The Green Pharmacy
HERBAL
HANDBOOK

Your **Comprehensive** Reference
to the Best Herbs for Healing

James A. Duke, Ph.D.

RODALE

REACH
™

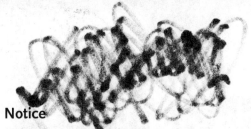

Notice

This book is intended as a reference volume only, not as a medical manual. The information given here is designed to help you make informed decisions about your health. It is not intended as a substitute for any treatment that may have been prescribed by your doctor. If you suspect that you have a medical problem, we urge you to seek competent medical help. Dosage options are descriptive only and not intended as prescriptive or recommended dosages.

Rodale/Reach is a trademark of Rodale Inc.

Printed in the United States of America on acid-free ∞, recycled paper ♺

Cover Designer: Laura Shaw
Interior Designer: Mark McGarry

Library of Congress Cataloging-in-Publication Data

Duke, James A., 1929–
    The green pharmacy herbal handbook : your comprehensive reference to
the best herbs for healing / James A. Duke
        p.   cm.
    Includes index.
    ISBN 1–57954–184–4 paperback
    1. Herbs—Therapeutic use—Handbooks, manuals, etc.   I. Title.
RM666.H33 D846 2000
615'.321—dc21   00–009941

Distributed to the book trade by St. Martin's Press

    4   6   8   10   9   7   5   paperback

Visit us on the Web at www.rodalebooks.com, or call us toll-free at (800) 848-4735.

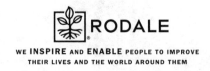

RODALE

WE **INSPIRE** AND **ENABLE** PEOPLE TO IMPROVE
THEIR LIVES AND THE WORLD AROUND THEM

In September 1975, I wrote my first article for *Organic Gardening* magazine. That was the beginning of an enjoyable, rewarding 25-year association with Rodale Inc., the Rodale family, and Rodale readers.

I dedicate this, my third book, to the publishing company, for Rodale's continuing efforts toward environmentally sound health and gardening and toward enlightening us all in farm, family, and "green farmacy."

I hope this book, designed to showcase the many benefits (and to admit the few shortcomings) of nature's most important green "farmaceuticals," will empower readers to find the right herbs to maintain, sustain, or regain their good health.

ACKNOWLEDGMENTS

This book was born at one of those far-flung trade shows—perhaps in Anaheim, Las Vegas, or San Antonio (after a while, they all look alike)—to promote my first Rodale book, *The Green Pharmacy*. I mentioned to a Rodale editor that I had a few more projects in the offing, including publication of my federally sponsored online database of medicinal herbs. Subsequent negotiations led to this popularized version of a most user-*unfriendly*, almost unreadable technical reference.

For the difficult task of translating that stilted, unwieldy database into an immediately understandable text, I thank Rodale editor Susan Clarey. I enjoyed our many lengthy e-mail exchanges and our more pleasant garden exchanges at my home. I also thank writer Joe Wargo for even more exchanges, via e-mail and, again more pleasantly, in the garden. Joe's enthusiasm for the project was sometimes greater than mine. He had to tone down my polemics on occasion, and I had to dampen his enthusiasm now and then. I think we both grew in the process.

Last, but no less important, I thank all the other people at Rodale who, for 25 years, have transformed this and my earlier sow's ears into publishable silk purses filled with the riches of our herbal heritage.

CONTENTS

The Green Pharmacy
HERBAL
HANDBOOK

PART ONE

Nature's Medicine Chest

We Americans like to think of ourselves as at the forefront of everything: technology, science, health care, business, culture. But for almost 2 decades, we've lagged far behind in at least one critical area: the search for new medicines. Or perhaps I should say a new search for old medicines.

Since the early 1980s, a high-powered, government-commissioned panel of top-notch authorities in Germany has been using high-tech scientific research to document the age-old therapeutic powers of medicinal plants—how they heal, why they heal, whether they heal, whether they pose any peril. The work of Commission E, as this group is called, now serves as a guideline for all of Europe in regulating the sale and dispensing of over-the-counter and prescription herbal medications (see "Commission E" on page 4).

THE UNITED STATES, never a notable player in searching for natural therapeutics, has no official equivalent to Commission E.

Welcome, therefore, to "Commission D," a maverick's guide to medicinal herbs, a loner's approach designed to serve as an authoritative yet down-to-earth American consumer's equivalent to the European effort. More idealistically, it's intended as a spur in the behind of the American medical establishment to undertake a wide-ranging comparative review of safer "farmaceutical" alternatives to often perilous synthetic drugs.

The "D" stands for Duke. That's me, the guy who was charged with finding, identifying, assessing, evaluating, classifying, and cataloging hundreds upon hundreds of potentially therapeutic plants for the U.S. Department of Agriculture's now-defunct Medicinal Plant Resources Laboratory. I headed the lab for but a brief five years, but I nurtured a passion for medicinal plants throughout my 29-year tenure as a botanist with the USDA.

Over those 3 decades, I foraged through jungles, rivers, and swamps the world over—Panama, Puerto Rico, Costa Rica, Mexico, Honduras, Guatemala, Ecuador, Chile, Bolivia, Peru, and elsewhere in South and Central America; China, Burma, India, Thailand, Vietnam, and Laos in Asia; Syria and Egypt in the Middle East; Kenya, Madagascar, São Tomé, and Tanzania in Africa.

I've rummaged around forests and fields in the United States, too, from boyhood homes in Alabama and North Carolina to the woods of my 6-acre home and Green Farmacy Garden in Maryland, where a microcosm of the world's medicinal flora now grows, largely untended but always lovingly watched.

Fortunately, I'm a chronic compiler. Early in my USDA years, I realized that the complexity of herbs is overwhelming and needed to be approached systematically, in a computerized database. I also believed that cataloging plant chemistry would provide a rationale for and explain many folk uses. It didn't take long for my database to assume a life of its own (see "Dr. Duke's Database: Medicine via Modem" on page 6).

The Green Pharmacy Herbal Handbook is a condensed, easy-to-read version of my full, highly technical compilation. It provides a concise but comprehensive look at almost 200 therapeutic plants, each graded in terms of medicinal efficacy and safety, all readily available at health food stores (and sometimes your local supermarket). It describes what the plants look like, explains their significance in the history of world civilizations, tells why they work, gives some commonly recommended dosages, and explains what (if any) side effects you should look for.

Commission E

In 1978, West Germany appointed a panel of experts to assess herbal medications. The group, called Commission E, operated under the direction of West Germany's Federal Institute for Drugs and Medical Devices. It examined more than 300 herbs and published its assessment of them in the German equivalent of the U.S. *Federal Register*, called the *Bundesanzeiger*.

Commission E is generally considered the preeminent governmental model for regulation and supervision of herbal supplements in the industrialized world. (The West Indies has a similar panel.) Its work is now the guideline for the European Union as it works toward a consistent set of rules governing the sale and dispensing of over-the-counter and prescription herbal medications.

Several American publishers have attempted to translate Commission E's work, some of them not very successfully. My vote for the best, most accurate translation (and excellent annotations) is the American Botanical Council's *Herbal Medicine: Expanded Commission E Monographs*, edited by Mark Blumenthal (executive director of the council), Alicia Goldberg, and Joel Brinckmann, published in 2000 by Integrative Medicine Communications, Newton, Massachusetts.

How to Use This Handbook

As befits an encyclopedic reference, the herbs in part two are arranged alphabetically. Each entry follows a precise format: name of herb, cursory description and history, therapeutic uses, medicinal properties, how it matches up against similarly acting synthetic drugs, dosage options, an overall safety rating, and possible problems and side effects.

So you can get the most out of the handbook, let me take you through an overview of each section.

Name

Each entry begins with the plant's most familiar common name. This may sound straightforward, but we could hit some snags along the way. For example, some people know black haw better as cramp bark. Others might not realize that melissa is more commonly called lemon balm. Where I think there might be some confusion, I've provided cross-references.

Following the common name is the scientific botanical name. The first part of the scientific name is the herb's genus, the classification right below its broader "family." The second part is its species, a narrower, more specific identification. A genus may contain only one or two species, or it may contain hundreds.

Sometimes the scientific name has become accepted as the common name. Melissa, for instance, is lemon balm's generic scientific name. Another example is coneflower. You won't find it among the other C herbs. It's amid the E herbs, under its scientific name of echinacea.

Individual species (and their sometimes almost infinite varieties) may look drastically different from each other or could be so similar as to tax the minds of the most knowledgeable botanical taxonomists. In cases where I think that few consumers or herbalists can distinguish among the species, I identify the plant by its genus and the catchall phrase "various species."

What It Is

Knowing an herb's common name and scientific name hardly does justice to the marvelously colorful diversity of our flora and the intimate extent to which human survival is entwined with the plant world. In this section, I try to provide a little of the plant's flavor—its looks, origins, and significance in human history.

Plants give us the very air we breathe. They supply most of our food, from the most exotic fruits and exquisite spices to the blandest staples—all able to sing a hundred different culinary choruses on one monotonous theme.

Until relatively recently, plants provided people with shelter, most of their clothing, and most of the dyes that colored their clothes. They have always been cultural, social, and religious symbols—from the lucky four-leaf clover

Dr. Duke's Database: Medicine via Modem

I started the publicly available federal database from which this book is derived in 1977 after being named chief of the Medicinal Plant Laboratory at the USDA. The lab may seem obscure, but it has a famous offspring. One of our main functions was an intensive worldwide search (for the National Cancer Institute) for herbs with anticancer potential. The global exploration eventually led to the creation of Taxol, a drug, known generically as paclitaxel, that's derived from various species of *Taxus*, better recognized as yew.

Since the beginning, my database has expanded far beyond its original scope. It now encompasses thousands of herbs and thousands of phytochemicals with possible therapeutic potential against almost any health problem. Fortunately, the USDA has continued to host the database beyond my retirement and beyond the closure of the Medicinal Plant Laboratory. I continue to update it regularly as new research trickles in. (One quite recent update, for instance, is that the same anticancer substance in yews has been found in hazelnuts. If verified, the discovery eventually could lead to a big price decrease in the cost of Taxol.)

Access to the full technical collection of medicinal herbs, including hundreds of other obscure plants not included in this book, is free and readily available to anyone with an Internet connection. Open up your Web browser and aim for:

www.ars-grin.gov/duke/
www.ars-grin.gov/duke/syllabus

You can search for herbs by name, by phytochemical, or by the conditions they address.

and George Washington's mythical cherry tree to the gap-toothed grin of a jack-o'-lantern and the kiss-me cluster of mistletoe hanging over a Yuletide doorway. They're sources of beauty, sources of recreation—and sources of medicine, let's not forget. We'll address that momentarily.

For those of us ever seeking the elusive truths of our universe, plants and the constantly endangered forests in which they thrive provide a restful and contemplative sanctuary. The forest is my living temple, and I hate to see it desecrated.

We know scientifically that plants communicate with each other, using some of the same chemicals that we now appropriate for medicinal purposes. When the bashful plant *(Mimosa pudica)* folds up its leaves, when the Venus's-flytrap *(Dionaea muscipula)* catches and engulfs an insect, when a touch-me-not *(Impatiens capensis)* ejaculates its seeds—are we seeing evidence of intelligence? When a stinging nettle *(Urtica dioica)* injects you with the same chemicals that course through your brain, is it trying to tell you something?

Do plants communicate with us? Do they have souls, as some people claim? I don't know. Perhaps we'll never know. But I have my suspicions.

Therapeutic Uses

For all herbs, any number of therapeutic claims have been made over the ages. Many have been verified scientifically. Others are supported by centuries of traditional use or by anecdotal accounts that have not been validated scientifically. This doesn't mean that such folk uses don't hold water. It means that science hasn't bothered to investigate and test these health-promoting claims. By contrast, because of either misinformation, misinterpretation, or outright deception motivated by greed, false claims have been made on behalf of many plants. Those claims have not withstood, or could not withstand, scientific scrutiny.

Medicinal Properties

How does the plant perform its therapeutic magic? What does it do inside your body? In attempting to answer these questions, scientists like to look for easy answers—one key to the closet, one piece to the puzzle, one phyto-chemical component. Nature is far more complex.

In this section, I try to explain why the herb works. Sometimes we know its physiologic effect; sometimes researchers have identified a specific phy-tochemical or group of phytochemicals thought to be responsible. I discour-age an emphasis on a single phytochemical answer—the silver bullet approach, as I call it. I prefer the multifaceted shotgun blast, and it's impor-tant to understand why.

The more you distill an herb down to one phytochemical essence, the more it resembles an unnatural, unbalanced drug capable of inflicting injury. (The silver-bullet mentality is responsible for why, to give you an example, so many bacteria are resistant to our drugs.) Probably even the most genetically simple alga contains thousands of phytochemicals, most of them working together to maintain that plant's health and survival. Perhaps

Key to Efficacy Ratings

I have devised a fair numerical rating system to assess each plant's medicinal value, based on my review of the research. Let me explain my leaf-based grad-ing system.

🌿🌿🌿 This is my highest score for therapeutic impact. A three-leaf rating means that the whole herb, as a food or whole-herb supplement, has proved itself in one or more strictly conducted scientific trials that involved people (not animals or petri dish cultures). This is "food farmacy" at its finest. Three leaves is a rigorous rating, not often seen in this book. Among those herbs that have earned the honor are bilberry, garlic, and saw palmetto.

🌿🌿 If an herbal extract or a major plant chemical (phytochemical, as it's called, with the prefix phyto meaning "plant-based") proved itself beneficial in research that involved people, it gets a two-leaf rating here. So does any thera-peutic use endorsed by Germany's Commission E. The lower rating isn't a shortchanging or downplaying of an herb's efficacy; it's a reflection of my fer-vent belief that we should not be trying to isolate silver bullets in nature's phar-macopeia. Any given leaf, root, or strip of bark contains thousands of phytochemical substances. They exist there for a reason—a reason that per-as many as 95 percent of those phytochemicals have at least one distinct purpose that benefits the plant—and sometimes the plant's predators (including you and me). For even the best-known herbs, we've only nibbled at the edges of identifying potentially useful compounds. Fewer than 5 percent of the plant world's members, in my estimation, have been studied extensively.

Most phytochemicals appear in a particular plant for an evolutionary reason that we may never understand. Any one of them could interact with any or all of the others—synergizing with one, inhibiting another. Remove one, and you might very well disrupt the entire synergistic concert.

We share with plants many of these biochemical compounds. You grew (as opposed to grew up with) these substances. Your genes have interacted with phytochemicals for millions of years. Long before you were born—even long before your ancestors were born—evolution ensured an affinity

haps we humans have yet to figure out. If we exclude them, we exclude them to our own possible detriment.

The two-leaf rating doesn't necessarily mean that the herbal extract is less medicinally effective than a three-leaf-rated whole herb. What it does mean is that to derive the intended therapeutic effect, you have to change the whole herb a bit, altering its phytochemical contents and their relative proportions.

One leaf means that an experiment not involving people showed some positive health effect. The study could have been done in a test tube or petri dish, or it could have involved lab mice or other animals. It could have focused on the whole herb, an extract, or an isolated phytochemical.

Folk Uses—This category is reserved for all unscientific, unsubstantiated health claims. They could be based on decades or centuries of folk use, on a large collection of case histories, or on anecdotal accounts. Folk applications may or may not work, although I tend to think that some validity must exist for a time-honored remedy. Keep in mind that many of yesterday's folk remedies are today's scientifically proven treatments.

between the biological processes in your body and the biochemicals in the plant world. You were meant to have many of them inside you. They're supposed to be there. That's why your body responds so positively to them, even in such tiny amounts. They're compensating for a deficiency, just as vitamin and mineral supplements do. (And let's not forget that herbs are often excellent sources of vitamins and minerals.)

Prescription Counterparts

Health insurance fraud, medical malpractice, and other such crimes generate big headlines, but just as heinous is the pitiful dearth of medical research into herbs, particularly research that rigorously compares the effectiveness of herbs with the effectiveness of currently favored pharmaceuticals for a given condition. In this section, you'll learn about some head-to-head studies, as well as about the best professional assessments of these herbs. Sometimes an herb works almost as well or just as well as a drug. At other times, the herb is the active ingredient in the medication. (At least a quarter of all our pharmaceuticals are derived from plants.) Occasionally, as with milk thistle and bilberry, the herb has no synthetic counterpart for certain indications.

Every year, a couple of herbs (or foods) kill a few people, usually because of insanely high dosages or unanticipated anaphylactic or allergic reactions. In the same year, properly prescribed, duly supervised drugs kill some 140,000 or so Americans. Hundreds of thousands of others suffer from and languish under myriad documented side effects of prescription and over-the-counter medications. And then there are the unanticipated reactions to insufficiently scrutinized new drugs.

Something's wrong here. Something needs to be righted.

I've dedicated much of my time to encouraging, persuading, and lobbying the American medical establishment, including the pharmaceutical industry, to conduct comparative studies of drugs and therapeutic herbs. I want to know what are the safest, most efficacious, most economical treatments for my family and me. I don't care if a treatment is natural, unnatural, or a hybrid of the two. Until head-to-head trials are conducted routinely, no one—not the doctor, the pharmacist, you, or me—knows conclusively whether a pharmaceutical is better than its herbal equivalent.

Some such research has been conducted, the bulk of it in Europe. And whenever a phytopharmaceutical has been tested against a medication, the herb often has proved itself to be a close therapeutic competitor and almost always safer, gentler, and less likely to cause side effects.

Often an herb doesn't give a pharmaceutical the full run for its money. Aside from a lack of research, that's one reason the "Prescription Counterparts" section does not appear in every entry. Instead, I often include a comment or a precaution that an herb "magnifies," "enhances," or "potentiates" the therapeutic actions of certain prescription medications.

I cannot prescribe; I'm a Ph.D., not an M.D. I must caution you to consult your physician if you are thinking about taking herbs along with prescription drugs. My personal opinion is that such cautions must be considered in context. If, for example, kava-kava enhances the effects of diazepam (Valium), should you not take the herb or should you take smaller dosages of the pharmaceutical? If St. John's wort potentiates some prescription antidepressants, should you shun the herb, which is free of side effects, and continue with full-strength dosages of the drug? Or should you ask your doctor to reduce or discontinue your drug dosages because you've found something that's safer, less likely to cause side effects, and less expensive?

You get the idea. Even if an herb isn't as potent as its prescription counterpart, it could help you minimize your reliance on the drug.

An important cautionary note here is that you must not adjust prescribed drug dosages on your own. Do so only after consulting with your physician. (An herbally enlightened doctor can do this intelligently and objectively.) Tell your doctor that you're tired of the prescription drug, its side effects, and its cost. Tell him or her that you want to take advantage of the demonstrated benefit that an herb offers. Show him or her this book or accounts of other research. And tell him or her that if the herb does have some benefit, you want a closely supervised reduction in your pharmaceutical dosages.

The notion will almost certainly be seen as controversial by most mainstream physicians and viewed skeptically. Don't feel intimidated. You probably know more about herbs than the average American doctor. Unlike in some European countries, U.S. medical schools do not require future physicians to study herbal medicine. The typical American doctor knows almost nothing about medicinal herbs.

Phyto Favorites

Which herbs do Americans take most? Here are the 13 bestsellers for 1998 in supermarkets, pharmacies, and other large retail stores. This list may not be a perfect reflection of today's herbal marketplace because it doesn't include sales from health food stores, mail-order outlets, health practitioners, and the Internet. Nevertheless, it is one good measure of trends in herb use.

1. Ginkgo biloba
2. St. John's wort
3. Ginseng
4. Garlic
5. Echinacea/goldenseal
6. Saw palmetto
7. Kava-kava
8. Pycnogenol/grape seed extract
9. Cranberry
10. Valerian
11. Evening primrose
12. Bilberry
13. Milk thistle

Ginkgo and St. John's wort were also the two bestsellers in Germany in 1996, but the rest of the list varies: (3) echinacea, (4) bromelain, (5) milk thistle, (6) mistletoe, (7) ivy, (8) stinging nettle, (9) saw palmetto, (10) myrtle, (11) hawthorn, (12) yeast, (13) horse chestnut.

Source: Mark Blumenthal, Alicia Goldberg, and Joel Brinckmann, eds., *Herbal Medicine: Expanded Commission E Monographs* (Newton, Mass.: Integrative Medicine Communications, 2000), pp. 475, 477.

Dosage Options

"How much should I take?" is an often-asked question that doesn't have a simple answer.

I never prescribe or recommend dosages. That's best left to an herb-savvy physician and to individual supplement manufacturers. In fact, whenever someone asks me how much of an herb to take, I steadfastly respond that he or she should follow the directions on the label.

Nevertheless, dosages do vary, based on the brand and on the herb's preparation. In this section, I list a number of different dosage ranges, all culled from labels and the professional and personal experience of others. How much you take depends on the form you use. You can eat the herb as a food, swallow it as an encapsulated supplement, drink it as a tea, put it under your tongue as a liquid extract or tincture, even apply it right to your skin. Let's take a look at your options.

Meals. Plants can be delicious, and "food farmacy" is my favorite way to self-medicate. For all herbs considered foods, feel free to use them as garnishes, spices, condiments, side dishes, or main courses.

Supplements. Most people don't have the luxury of going out into the backyard and getting herbs straight from the garden. Although I grow my own herbs on my 6-acre Green Farmacy plot, I still, more often than not, take standardized supplemental extracts of certain therapeutic plants. Some authorities disagree, but I believe that the best way to make sure you're getting a measurable, consistent amount of a given active ingredient is to take a standardized supplement.

Plants vary wildly in their phytochemical content—depending on the species, processing, handling, harvesting, fertilizer, weather, garden, pests, and gardener. A consistent potency is usually best to ensure a consistent medicinal effect. That's what the process of standardization does. It ensures that you get a specific amount of one or more of the major phytochemicals. Because you know you're getting specific amounts of their phytochemicals, they're more medicinally reliable.

I wouldn't standardize coffee into a couple of capsules of caffeine. I wouldn't want to standardize an onion. But I would prefer standardized versions of many other herbs.

Some brands of standardized extracts are great; some are almost devoid of important ancillary components and synergistic phytochemicals. How do you know you're picking a good one? The clues are on the label or a package insert. Here's what to look for.

- Proper identification of the herb's scientific name
- Identification of the major phytochemical for which the supplement is standardized, including the percentage of the major active ingredient
- A list of ancillary ingredients
- A specific dosage recommendation (If no dosage is listed, choose another brand.)
- An expiration date, because potency declines over time

- An address and a toll-free number for any questions or complaints
- A list of side effects, drug interactions, and reasons why you should not or might not want to take the herb.

Standardized supplements may cost more, but their guaranteed potency is often worth it. The dosages you'll see in this book are representative of what you'll find on better brands in health food stores. Use them as a guide but stick with what the label recommends. Sometimes I also note the equivalent dosage (usually a lot higher) for unstandardized supplements.

Teas. Few things are more refreshing, relaxing, or enjoyable than a cup of herbal tea. Your body requires fluid, and an herbal tea is a pleasant way to dispense medicine and provide fluid.

You won't always be able to use a tea bag. You may have to use loose leaves (usually a teaspoon or two of the dried herb) that you'll have to filter out of the tea. (Or try using a tea ball.) For herbs and flowers, you should let them steep in hot water for anywhere from 5 to 20 minutes. That's called an infusion. For roots, stems, and bark, you have to boil them in water for the same period of time, maybe more. That's called a decoction.

Tinctures. Tinctures are alcohol- or vinegar-based versions of teas. Sometimes they're stronger than teas; sometimes they're not. It's easiest to buy a tincture at a health food store, but if you're ambitious, you can make your own. Just dump a lot of the fresh or dried herb (there are no precise measurements) into a jar containing vodka or vinegar and let it steep for anywhere from 2 days to 2 weeks or more. Tinctures are especially good at capturing volatile compounds from aromatic herbs.

Poultices and compresses. Sometimes the best internal medicine is applied externally. When applicable, you might benefit from a poultice, a clump of the herb, usually moistened, that's put directly to the skin. Or, if the herb is unwieldy or messy, you might want to first warp it in some cheesecloth or another thin cloth, perhaps also taping it to your body. You also could apply a compress, which is just a cloth soaked in an herbal tea, tincutre, or liquid extract.

Essential oils. I do not advocate ingesting the uncut, aromatic, essential oils of plants. Instead, I advise *diluting them significantly before ingesting*. Swallowing them straight—sometimes merely inhaling them by a small child—can be dangerous, perhaps fatal. Applying them full strength to your skin also can cause problems. To minimize the chance of a skin reaction, always dilute the oil in your bathwater or in an innocuous carrier substance such as almond oil, evening primrose oil, olive oil, vegetable oil, or rubbing alcohol.

Note: Occasionally, dosages of herbs may differ depending on what condition you're trying to treat. I'll let you know about this. I'll also address other considerations—such as when to take the herb, what to take it with, or how to offset an unpleasant taste—when pertinent.

Safety Rating

Around Thanksgiving about a decade ago, the FDA called me to report a man dead in a car that was loaded with mugwort *(Artemisia vulgaris)*, an herb used ceremonially by Native Americans and Chinese and as a condiment and flavoring agent in parts of Europe and Asia. The FDA official wanted to know what toxins mugwort might contain. After consulting my database, I responded that one phytochemical, thujone, could, in exceedingly large dosages, cause convulsions. I also dutifully reported that thujone was a main phytochemical in absinthe, the addictive, brain-deteriorating alcoholic drink thought to have driven Vincent van Gogh mad.

Alarmed by the possible connection between the cadaver and the plant, the agency official hinted that perhaps mugwort should be banned. I had to point out that if the FDA banned mugwort, it would also, in all fairness, have to ban sage *(Salvia officinalis)*, an indispensable Thanksgiving seasoning that can contain even more thujone than mugwort.

Ban sage and . . . there goes the turkey stuffing!

I never heard from the FDA again, and I never found out what actually killed that poor man. I do know, though, that mugwort wasn't banned, nor was sage. I suppose I could brag that I single-handedly saved a savory Thanksgiving for America, but there's a larger, more serious point to my tale: All compounds, whether natural or manmade, have safe, active, toxic, and lethal levels. Each and every chemical in you, me, and a carob tree probably can, in a sufficiently high concentration, kill us.

Thanks to nature's wisdom, though, few plant chemicals appear in amounts sufficient to cause alarm. In other words, virtually every herb, if

Key to Safety Ratings

Each herbal entry in this book is graded as to whether I think it's safer than coffee, equally as safe as coffee, or almost as safe as coffee. A rating of:

3 means that I think the herb is safer than coffee.

2 means that the herb poses no more of a risk to your well-being than does a cup of java.

1 means that the herb likely presents more of a risk than does coffee but is still okay to use.

Only a few herbs carry a "do not use" rating. Even though some of them are readily available at health food stores and elsewhere, I don't advocate their use in any form or any amount. They may not kill you, but they could pose serious risks.

If you're worried about any health hazards associated with coffee, you should be equally worried about all the other herbs I've rated 2 or 1. Some people are more sensitive to coffee (and other herbs) than others. Where equally efficacious options are available, you should opt for an herb with a 2 rating over one with a 1 rating. You can approach herbs with a 3 rating with even less trepidation. Personally, I wouldn't think twice about recommending that my 120-pound daughter drink three cups a day of a tea made from an herb with a 3 rating, two cups of a tea made with an herb with a 2 rating, and one cup of a tea made with an herb with a 1 rating.

(Incidentally, mugwort, though not in this book, gets a rating of 1 in my on-line database, not because a carload can kill you but because a carload might induce an abortion. Sage, in contrast, earns a rating of 3, although a carload of it, too, might induce an abortion, not to mention horribly over-seasoned turkey dressing. Stick with reasonable amounts, and you'll be fine.)

used in an appropriate manner, can be used safely with no major cause for concern. Could sage kill you? Maybe, but I doubt that you could ingest enough of it at one time to get the job done.

The Coffee Connection

The concept of safety is relative. Some herbs are safer than others; some pose a greater likelihood of physiologic reactions that may not be totally desirable. Even the most innocuous of substances is going to induce an idiosyncratic reaction in someone somewhere in the world. (Peanuts kill about two Americans annually from anaphylactic shock.)

To give an immediately recognizable reference point for the relative safety of these plants, I've used as a benchmark the most frequently ingested herbal drug of all in the U.S.—coffee. Few people, herbal newcomers and longtime herbal nitpickers alike, realize that coffee is medicinal. Straight caffeine is a drug; coffee, the beverage, is what's termed a "dilute drug," just like any other herbal tea. Talk to a chemist, and you'll learn that caffeine has an oral "LD50" of 192. This technical lingo means that it takes 192 milligrams of caffeine to kill one-half of a group of experimental rats that weigh 2.2 pounds (1 kilogram) each. (LD stands for "lethal dose.") Translated into human proportions, that means it would take 21,120 milligrams of pure, isolated caffeine—all ingested in one short sitting—to kill me, a 242-pound experimental rat. The average cup of coffee contains anywhere from 10 to 100 milligrams of caffeine. I like my coffee, but I don't drink between 200 and 2,000 cups in one sitting.

Chemists and pharmacists have calculated an LD50 for just about everything. Most herbs possess an LD50 that is orders of magnitude safer than that of caffeine, and even full-strength essential oils have safer LD50s than pure caffeine. I have not cited LD50s in this book (they're in that more technical online database of mine), but I've incorporated the calculations into my own rating system.

Precautions

Just as all substances have safe, toxic, and lethal levels, all medications (whether synthetic pharmaceuticals, whole herbs, standardized concentrates of whole herbs, or isolates of herbs) have effects on the body. As noted previously, FDA-approved drugs kill an estimated 140,000 Americans every year and afflict hundreds of thousands more with adverse effects that range from irksome to intolerable, from temporary to irreversible.

A couple of herbs might do that, too, but not many. As I've said, your genes know these herbal compounds more intimately than they know synthetic pharmaceuticals. Your genes may not yet know the drugs that were

The Seven Most Studied Herbs

Thousands of animal and test tube experiments have been performed on herbs, but practical, clinical research lags far behind. Here are Germany's seven most studied herbs, whose therapeutic benefits have been verified in studies on people. The rankings are based on research conducted as far back as the late 1970s and as recently as 1997.

Some herbs have been the subject of more clinical studies, while others, though less frequently examined, have been tested on more people. I list them here alphabetically, followed by the number of studies and the total number of people involved.

Herb	Number of Studies	Number of People
Garlic	18	2,920
Ginkgo biloba	36	2,326
Hawthorn	13	791
Horse chestnut	8	798
Kava	6	469
St. John's wort	22	1,851
Valerian	8	560

Source: Mark Blumenthal, Alicia Goldberg, and Joel Brinckmann, eds., *Herbal Medicine: Expanded Commission E Monographs* (Newton, Mass.: Integrative Medicine Communications, 2000), p. 478; citing, in part, V. Schulz et al. *Rational Phytotherapy* (New York: Springer, 1998)

created 2 months, 2 years, or 2 decades ago, and they certainly don't know the drugs that will be invented tomorrow. That's why, on average, phytochemicals, even if isolated, are less likely than drugs to upset the equilibrium of the hundreds of homeostatic reactions in the body. This section tells you whether there is cause for concern.

Everything in Moderation

Although few of the phytochemicals in herbs rated 1, 2, or 3 appear in quantities sufficient to provoke alarm, their mere presence sends up a red flag in some quarters. Black pepper and basil contain safrole, which, when isolated and administered in huge doses, can cause cancer in people with weak immune systems. The potentially allergenic pollens and sesquiterpenes in artichokes, chamomile, and echinacea could, in sufficiently large amounts, provoke an anaphylactic reaction in sensitive people. The menthol in peppermint, spearmint, and dozens of other plants (even sunflower oil) can cause kidney failure and even kill a baby—again in ridiculously large dosages. The tannins in tea and other herbs supposedly can cause liver damage and throat cancer. Yet these are the same tannins in the same green and black tea that so much research shows actually prevent cancer.

What does all this mean? First, too much of anything isn't good. Second, somebody, somewhere, may be more susceptible to a substance's effects, good or bad, than everyone else.

Most of using herbs medicinally is just plain common sense. Don't take ludicrously large dosages; many herbs, while generally safe in the therapeutic amounts suggested on supplement labels, are not always harmless in big dosages. Also, be certain you don't confuse herbal effects. If you have diarrhea, for instance, you really shouldn't ingest an herb that's known as a laxative, no matter what its other therapeutic properties. If you have a problem with blood coagulation, don't take an herb known for thinning the blood. If you have an autoimmune disorder, don't ingest an herb known to bolster the immune system that is turning against you. If you're pregnant, don't consume an herb with a reputation for stimulating uterine contractions.

We're All Different

If even a few people have reacted unfavorably to an herb, I'll tell you here. Everyone's different physiologically, and some people are just more sensitive than others. Some people will be able to take larger dosages than others, too.

Essential Oils

As noted previously, stay away from ingesting pure essential oils. If you want to try them topically, always dilute them. And keep the oils away from infants and children; inhaling even a few drops can kill a baby.

Drug Interactions

If you're taking a drug whose effects an herb might exaggerate or negate, make sure you read this part of the entry. As mentioned previously, if an

If You Are Pregnant

In 1998, President Bill Clinton beseeched pharmaceutical companies to include children and babies in their studies of drug safety. They rebuffed him, complaining about costs and other difficulties in compiling such data on children. Therefore, very few prescription or over-the-counter drugs can claim to be safe for pregnant women and nursing moms. Yet some pregnant women and nursing mothers do take these medications. Why should herbal medicines be held to a higher standard?

Yet most so-called experts (even generally pro-herb people) warn against using various plants if you're pregnant, planning to get pregnant, or nursing a newborn. Those warnings appear sparingly on these pages, for a few reasons. First, if you're pregnant or lactating, you must go far out of your way to be careful about everything you and your child ingest—not only herbal supplements but also foods and, above all, prescription and over-the-counter drugs. Herbs work like drugs. They should be included in a pregnant or nursing woman's concerns.

If you're pregnant or nursing and you or your baby need medicine for a problem, don't blindly follow advice not to take herbs. Instead, seek your physician's or pediatrician's help in comparing the benefits and risks of all possible treatments, synthetic and natural. Depending on the circumstances, pick either the safest one or the one with the best risk-benefit ratio.

If any pregnancy-related or pediatric concerns exist, you'll read about them in this section.

herb magnifies the action of a drug, don't shy away from it automatically. Look at it as a possible means to decrease your dependence on the pharmaceutical. You might be able to wean yourself off the drug entirely or get by on smaller dosages. Don't do so on your own, though. Again, recruit the help of your doctor (preferably one well-schooled in herbal medicine) to assess all possible risks and benefits of all possible treatments.

Preferable Prescriptions?

For many common health problems and complaints, an herbal alternative exists for the prescription or over-the-counter counterpart that doctors so often recommend and prescribe. Following are some of the main contenders, categorized by ailment. Not all potentially helpful herbs are listed for each condition, just those natural "Davids" that have displayed the most competitive promise as alternatives to the pharmaceutical "Goliaths." See the individual entries for referrals to herbal combinations that may magnify the therapeutic results.

Remember that you should not try to treat serious health problems on your own. Nor should you stop taking any prescribed medication without first consulting with your doctor.

Use this list only as a starting point for further investigation—again, in conjunction with your doctor, who, in a perfect world, would be a physician trained in and knowledgeable about herbal medicine. Talk to your doctor about how herbal medicine can play a role in maintaining your good health or in your return to full health.

CONDITION	HERB	PHARMACEUTICAL
Acne	Tea tree, calendula	Benzoyl peroxide (Oxy 10), tretinoin (Retin-A), tetracycline
Alcoholism	Kudzu, evening primrose	Disulfiram (Antabuse)
Allergies	Chamomile, nettle	Corticosteroids, antihistamines
Alzheimer's disease	Ginkgo, rosemary, sage	Tacrine (Cognex)
Angina (chest pains)	Hawthorn, willow	Beta-blockers, nitroglycerin
Anxiety	Kava-kava, hops, passionflower, valerian	Diazepam (Valium), alprazolam (Xanax), lorazepam (Ativan), clonazepam (Klonopin), paroxetine hydrochloride (Paxil)
Arrhythmia (irregular heart rhythm)	Hawthorn	Verapamil (Calan)
Arthritis	Cayenne, celery seed, evening primrose, ginger, turmeric, willow	Acetaminophen, corticosteroids, nonsteroidal anti-inflammatory drugs (NSAIDs)

(continued)

Preferable Prescriptions? (cont.)

CONDITION	HERB	PHARMACEUTICAL
Athlete's foot	Garlic, tea tree oil	Griseofulvin (Grisactin, Fulvicin)
Boils	Tea tree oil	Erythromycin
Breast cancer	Red clover, soy	Raloxoifen (Evista), Tamoxifen (Nolvadex)
Bronchitis	Echinacea, elderberry	Atropine, dextromethorphan, codeine
Burns	Aloe	Silver sulfadiazine (Silvadene cream)
Bursitis, tendinitis	Licorice	Hydrocortisone
Canker sores	Goldenseal	Ambesol
Cirrhosis	Milk thistle	No comparable drug
Colds	Echinacea, elderberry, boneset	Decongestants, acetaminophen, over-the-counter cold remedies
Colitis	Peppermint, psyllium	Sulfasalazine (Azulfidine)
Constipation	Cascara sagrada, psyllium, senna	Ex-Lax (which now contains senna), other prescription and over-the-counter laxatives
Cuts, scrapes	Tea tree oil	Mercurochrome, iodine, antiseptics
Cystitis	Bearberry, cranberry	Trimethoprim and sulfamethoxazole (Bactrim), phenazopyridine hydrochloride (Pyridium), antibiotics
Depression	St. John's wort	Fluoxetine hydrochloride (Prozac), amitriptyline hydrochloride (Elavil), trazadone hydrochloride (Trazadone), sertraline hydrochloride (Zoloft), monoamine oxidase inhibitors (MAOIs)
Diarrhea	Bilberry, raspberry	Imodium, Lomotil, Kaopectate
Diverticulitis	Peppermint	Penicillin, erythromycin

Condition	Herb	Pharmaceutical
Earache	Echinacea, garlic, goldenseal	Decongestants
Eczema	Chamomile, evening primrose	Hydrocortisone cream, corticosteroids
Eye infections	Goldenseal	Antibiotics, chloramphenicol (Chloromycetin), sulfacetamide (Sultrin)
Flu	Echinacea, elderberry	Acetaminophen, over-the-counter cold remedies
Fungal infections	Garlic	Nystatin (Mycostatin), other antifungal drugs
Gas	Fennel, rosemary	Gaviscon; such simethicone-containing products as Maalox and Mylanta
Gout	Celery seed	Allopurinol
Hair loss (male pattern baldness)	Saw palmetto	Finasteride (Propecia), minoxidil (Rogaine)
Hay fever	Nettle	Antihistamines, pseudoephedrine, decongestants
Heart disease	Hawthorn	Digitalis, many other medications
Hemorrhoids	Butcher's broom, horse chestnut, witch hazel	Preparation H, Tucks
Hepatitis	Milk thistle	Interferon (Roferon-A)
Herpes	Lemon balm	Acyclovir (Zovirax)
High blood pressure	Garlic, celery seed, onion, beans	Beta-blockers, angiotensin converting enzyme (ACE) inhibitors, diuretics
High blood sugar	Fenugreek, gymnema, garlic, bitter melon	Insulin, metformin (Glucophage), other oral diabetes drugs, such as the many sulfonylureas

(continued)

Preferable Prescriptions? (cont.)

CONDITION	HERB	PHARMACEUTICAL
High cholesterol/atherosclerosis	Garlic, gugul, soy	Lovastatin (Mevacor), simvastatin (Zocar), atorvastatin (Lipitor), various vasodilators
Hyperthyroidism	Bugle	Radiation exposure, thyroid hormone replacement
Infections	Garlic, tea tree oil	Erythromycin, other antibiotics and antiseptics
Indigestion	Anise, fennel, peppermint, ginger, chamomile	Famotidine (Pepcid), other antacids
Insomnia	Kava-kava, hops, lemon balm, evening primrose, valerian	Triazolam (Halcion), diazepam (Valium), other sedatives and over-the-counter sleep aids
Intermittent claudication	Ginkgo, garlic	Pentoxiphylline (Trental)
Irritable bowel syndrome	Chamomile, psyllium	Chlordiazepoxide hydrochloride and clidinium bromide (Librax), Donnatal
Labor delay	Black cohosh, blue cohosh	Oxytocin (Pitocin)
Menopause	Black cohosh, red clover, soy extracts, dong quai	Hormone replacement therapy
Migraine	Feverfew	Sumatriptan (Imitrex), Verapamil (Calan)
Morning sickness	Ginger	Various over-the-counter products
Motion sickness	Ginger	Scopolamine (Donnatal), Dramamine
Mushroom poisoning	Milk thistle	No comparable pharmaceutical
Night blindness	Bilberry, blueberry	No comparable pharmaceutical
Premenstrual tension and cramps	Buchu, chasteberry, kava-kava, red clover, soy, raspberry, evening primrose	Naproxen (Naprosyn), NSAIDs, diuretics, analgesics

Condition	Herb	Pharmaceutical
Prostate enlargement (noncancerous)	Evening primrose, saw palmetto, nettle, pumpkin	Finasteride (Proscar), terazosin hydrochloride (Hytrin)
Psoriasis	Licorice	Hydrocortisone cream
Retinopathy	Bilberry, blueberry	No pharmaceutical equivalent
Shingles	Cayenne	Acyclovir (Zovirax), famciclovir (Famvir)
Stress	Kava-kava, hops, passionflower, valerian	Diazepam (Valium), alprazolam (Xanax), lorazepam (Ativan), clonazepam (Klonopin), paroxetine hydrochloride (Paxil)
Tinnitus	Ginkgo	Corticosteroids
Toothache	Willow, clove	Ibuprofen, aspirin
Ulcers	Licorice, aloe	Antacids, beta-blockers, cimetidine (Tagamet), ranitidine hydrochloride (Zantac)
Yeast infections	Garlic, black walnut, tea tree oil	Clotrimazole (Lotrimin), Nystatin, miconazole nitrate (Mycostatin), ketoconazole (Nizoral)

PART TWO

HERBS FOR HEALING

Herbs in this section are arranged alphabetically for easy reference. Each entry follows a uniform format: name of herb, description and history, therapeutic uses, medicinal properties, prescription counterparts (where applicable), dosage options, safety rating, and precautions including possible side effects.

For a more detailed explanation of the therapeutic uses, safety ratings, and other information contained in each entry, see How to Use This Handbook, p. 5.

ALFALFA *(Medicago sativa)*

What It Is:
A widely cultivated herbaceous legume that can be grown just about anywhere, alfalfa came from Europe, but it's been naturalized all over North America, particularly in the western states. It's been a longtime food staple for cattle and horses the world over, but it's also sprouted a good reputation among salad lovers. Alfalfa sprouts, sans the purple yellow flowers that bloom on a fully grown plant, are a staple at salad bars and in the produce section of almost any grocery store.

Therapeutic Uses:
🐾 Diabetes, high cholesterol, indigestion, menopause, water retention, yeast infections.
▦ Folk uses: Alcoholism, arthritis, asthma, bad breath, cancer, hay fever, inflammation, prostatitis, peptic ulcers, rheumatism.

Medicinal Properties:
Alfalfa contains plant world equivalents of human estrogens, so a woman, whether she's going through menopause or breastfeeding a baby, may derive some benefit from it. The plant's manganese content might help people with diabetes control high blood sugar. Chemicals called saponins can help lower blood cholesterol (by impeding intestinal absorption) without affecting heart-healthy high-density lipoprotein (HDL) cholesterol.

Dosage Options:
Alfalfa sprouts contain nutrients, but the leaves, science suggests, contain the best healing potential. A typical dosage is three or four 370-milligram capsules of alfalfa leaves three times a day or 15 to 30 drops of alfalfa tincture four times a day, or a tea using 1 to 2 teaspoons of dried alfalfa leaves in a cup of boiling water; drink up to three times a day.

Safety Rating: 1

Precautions:
In small, reasonable amounts, alfalfa causes no known side effects or problems. If you eat upwards of 120 grams of seeds a day, you might notice some abdominal discomfort, flatulence, and diarrhea. Because of a toxic amino acid called canavanine, long-term consumption of high dosages of alfalfa seeds or sprouts could trigger a

recurrence of systemic lupus erythematosus in people previously treated for the condition. If you have lupus or are in remission, you shouldn't consume alfalfa seeds.

ALOE *(Aloe vera)*

What It Is:
With its fleshy, fingerlike leaves, this African-based member of the lily family is arguably one of the best known of all herbal remedies, with a reputation spanning at least the past 2,000 years. The succulent perennial grows in sandy soil in any dry, sunny place, including on windowsills. It is useful for cuts, scrapes, burns, and other minor skin injuries. Do not confuse aloe vera gel with products made from the juice of the dried inner leaves (see "Aloes" on page 29).

Therapeutic Uses:
∾ Abrasions, arthritis, asthma, bedsores, bronchitis, bruises, bug bites, burns, dermatitis, dry skin, frostbite, mouth ulcers, peptic ulcers, radiation burns, ringworm, wounds.

▓ Folk uses: Acne, anemia, blindness, coughing, diabetes, dry eyes, eczema, glaucoma, hemorrhoids, psoriasis, seborrhea, sunburn, syphilis, vaginitis.

Medicinal Properties:
The gel from freshly snapped leaves apparently soothes pain by dilating the capillaries, thus stimulating better blood flow to burned or wounded skin. It also encourages healing to occur between tissue cells. A tonic and other supplements made from the gel are said to aid digestion.

Dosage Options:
Preservative-pumped commercial aloe shampoos and skin care products (containing stabilized aloe) rarely, if ever, pack the therapeutic punch of fresh aloe. Avoid them. Get a plant, put it on a windowsill, water it every once in a while, and wait for the next minor emergency. Aloe vera requires very little care and virtually no plant know-how. When you cut yourself, burn a finger on the stove, or sit out in the sun too long, simply snap off one of the lower leaves, slice it lengthwise, and coat the wound with the gooey gel.

Safety Rating: 2

Precautions:
Do not confuse aloe vera gel with aloe products made from the leaf's inner juices (see the next entry). The gel and products made from it are entirely safe.

ALOES; DRUG ALOE *(Aloe vera)*

What It Is:
Aloes, or drug aloe, made from the juice (not the gel) of the dried inner leaves, is a strong laxative.

Therapeutic Uses:
🐛🐛 Constipation.
▨ Folk uses: Atherosclerosis, colic, high blood sugar, infections, lack of menstruation, liver problems, menstrual irregularities, seborrhea, tuberculosis, tumors, ulcers, worms.

Medicinal Properties:
At one time, aloes was a widely used laxative, but not anymore. The anthraquinones in drug aloe are a little too strong. They work, but they're among the last resorts to remedy constipation. First, eat a high-fiber diet. For supplemental help, turn to psyllium or cascara sagrada (see "Psyllium" on page 178 and "Cascara Sagrada" on page 63).

Dosage Options:
250 milligrams of aloe juice in capsule form or 50 to 200 milligrams of the dried juice per day.

Safety Rating: 1

Precautions:
Certainly not for long-term use. You might get abdominal pains and gastrointestinal irritation. Don't take it if you have hemorrhoids or kidney disease. The gel and the dried-leaf juice are two entirely different things. You have nothing to worry about if you stick with the gel from freshly cut aloe leaves. But if you ingest a product containing aloes, better clear a path to the bathroom for the next 6 hours or so.

ANISE *(Pimpinella anisum)*

What It Is:
With its feathery leaves and clusters of small yellow or white flowers, anise grows throughout North America, usually in gardens and, every once in a while, in the wild. The leaves can be used as a garnish or added to salads. The brown fruit, which looks more like a seed, contains the essential oil that serves as the licorice-tasting spice found in candies, cough nostrums, and ouzo.

Therapeutic Uses:
🐛🐛 Bronchitis, colds, coughing, fever, gallbladder problems, liver problems, poor appetite, sore throat.

🐛 Anemia, bad breath, breast milk deficiency, colic, gas, indigestion, psoriasis.

▥ Folk uses: Congestion, cramps, low libido, male menopause, morning sickness, nausea, scabies.

Medicinal Properties:
The therapeutic powers of anise's phytochemicals, including creosol and alpha-pinene, are so apparent and well-established that the herb is commonly used in preparations that break up congestion, ease coughing, and relieve gas. Another constituent, anethole, is similar in chemical structure to the stress hormones adrenaline and noradrenaline, and it is thought to encourage the secretion of breast milk.

Dosage Options:
Pour a cup of boiling water over 1 to 2 teaspoons of crushed aniseeds, steep for 10 to 15 minutes, strain, and enjoy. Have a cup in the morning and then again in the evening. Alternatively, a typical dosage is ½ to 1 teaspoon of anise tincture three times a day.

Safety Rating: 2

Precautions:
A few people might experience an allergic response to anise, particularly dermatologic, respiratory, or gastrointestinal reactions. In reasonable amounts, though, most people will be fine. If you try anise oil, don't take too much; as little as 1 to 5 milliliters could cause nausea, seizures, vomiting, and a buildup of fluid in the lungs.

ARTICHOKE *(Cynara cardunculus)*

What It Is:
One of the oldest and most commonly cultivated vegetables, this herbaceous plant is known for its large, edible, thistlelike flower heads.

Therapeutic Uses:
🐛🐛 Gallbladder problems, indigestion, poor appetite.

🐛 Arsenic poisoning, atherosclerosis, blood clotting, constipation, flatulence, high blood sugar, high cholesterol, high triglycerides, high uric acid, inflammation, jaundice, kidney problems, liver problems, nausea, tumor growth, water retention.

▥ Folk uses: Anemia, arthritis, dropsy, gallstones, gout, insufficient urination, itching, low libido, rheumatism, snakebite.

Medicinal Properties:
Cynarin and other compounds can stimulate bile secretion from the gallbladder, thus aiding digestion. Animal experiments have shown that artichoke phytochemicals also help detoxify and regenerate the liver. Small clinical trials involving people have produced mixed results on the question of whether artichoke can reduce blood fats; some studies have shown a beneficial effect, but others have not.

Dosage Options:
Enjoy pickled and cooked artichokes first, then turn to supplements. Possible amounts include two or three 100-milligram capsules, each standardized for 15 milligrams of caffeoylquinic acids, every day; 1 to 4 grams of artichoke leaves three times a day; or ½ to 2 teaspoons of a liquid extract daily.

Safety Rating: 3

Precautions:
A few overly sensitive people might be allergic to artichoke extracts, developing a rash or another dermatologic reaction.

ASHWAGANDA *(Withania somniferum)*

What It Is:
A member of the nightshade family, ashwaganda is native to India but now is also grown in the United States. It's often touted as the Indian version of ginseng, given its use in Ayurvedic medicine as an all-purpose tonic. Traditional Ayurvedic physicians prescribed preparations of the plant's roots for everything from hiccups to a variety of gynecologic concerns. What we now know is that the plant helps articularly as a mild sedative, an anti-inflammatory for creaky joints, and a libido booster.

Therapeutic Uses:
🍂 Alzheimer's disease, anemia, arthritis, asthma, cancer, erectile dysfunction, herpes, high cholesterol, high fever, inflammation, leukocytosis, low libido, lung cancer, morphine addiction, ringworm, stress, syphilis, ulcers.

▨ Folk uses: Backache, bronchitis, carbuncles, eye inflammation, convulsions, cramps, dermatitis, diarrhea, hemorrhoids, high blood pressure, immune system problems, insomnia, lumbago, nausea, prostatitis, rheumatism, sores, swelling, tuberculosis, tumors.

Medicinal Properties:
In the Ayurvedic medicine of India, ashwaganda is regarded as a general all-purpose tonic, good for just about anything that ails you. Research shows that its active ingredients, called withanolides, may bolster the immune system, buck up stamina,

fight inflammation and infections, oppose tumors, reduce stress, revive libido, protect the liver, and soothe savaged nerves.

Dosage Options:
150 to 600 milligrams of a standardized extract every day. You could also take 2 to 3 grams of powdered ashwaganda root daily or drink a cup of tea made by pouring boiling water over 5 teaspoons of the dried herb every day.

Safety Rating: 1

Precautions:
Stick with the standardized extract or the powdered herb; eating the berries might cause severe gastrointestinal pain. Ashwaganda also might heighten the effects of pharmaceutical barbiturates.

ASTRAGALUS *(Astragalus membranaceous)*

What It Is:
Native to northeastern China, where it's known as *huang qi* (yellow leader), this perennial is a member of the pea family. Medicinally, its long, fibrous roots are the Asian equivalent of echinacea.

Therapeutic Uses:
  Angina, colds, kidney problems.
  Autoimmune disorders, cancer, cervical inflammation, chronic fatigue syndrome, diabetes, encephalitis, fatigue, flu, heart problems, herpes, high blood pressure, HIV, immune system problems, infections, infertility, inflammation, low white blood cell count, side effects of chemotherapy, sore throat, ulcers, viral hepatitis.
  Folk uses: Diarrhea, fever, lack of appetite, myocarditis, palpitations, paralysis, postdelivery problems, prolapse, uterine pain.

Medicinal Properties:
An antiviral, antibacterial, and anti-inflammatory, astragalus fortifies the immune system on several levels, including, perhaps, by increasing the body's production of interferon. Nasal sprays and oral ingestion have protected lab mice from parainfluenza virus type 1. Other animal experiments have found some evidence that astragalus protects against the common cold, reduces water retention, and lowers high blood sugar and high blood pressure. One study on people found that taking 200 milligrams of astragalus root extract for every 2.2 pounds of body weight increased urine output by 64 percent and sodium excretion by 14.5 percent.

Dosage Options:
1,500 to 3,000 milligrams in divided doses, 2 to 30 grams of astragalus root, ½ to 1 teaspoon of a tincture, or 1 teaspoon to 1 tablespoon of a liquid extract daily.

Safety Rating: 2

Precautions:
None reported. Just don't pick your own out in the wild; some species are toxic.

BASIL *(Ocimum basilicum)*

What It Is:
A member of the mint family, basil is an aromatic annual herb. The plant, which may grow as tall as 2 to 3 feet, sprouts tiny white or purple-tinged flowers. Its leaves—sometimes green, sometimes purplish; sometimes smooth-edged, sometimes serrated—give off their characteristic scent when bruised.

Therapeutic Uses:
🍃 Acne, bug bites, gas, dental problems, parasitic infections, wounds.
▦ Folk uses: Alcoholism, arthritis, bruises, chills, colds, constipation, cramps, depression, heart problems, indigestion, itching, nausea, pain, rheumatism, ringworm, snakebite, sore throat, swelling, warts.

Medicinal Properties:
Basil contains many antiviral compounds, which no doubt is why it's a time-honored folk remedy for warts. Other phytochemicals might fight plaque formation on teeth.

Dosage Options:
For a natural insect repellent, just rub some crushed leaves on your skin. To kill a wart, rub leaves on the nub daily and cover with a bandage. Or, steep 1 to 2 teaspoons of the dried herb in a cup of water or take ½ to 1 teaspoon of basil tincture up to three times a day.

Safety Rating: 2

Precautions:
As a spice in pasta sauce and other foods, basil is entirely safe. But the essential oil from basil contains a chemical called estragole, which might cause cancer in extremely large doses.

BAYBERRY *(Myrica cerifera)*

What It Is:
The leaves of this shrub, which grows near swamps and marshes along Lake Erie and the Atlantic coast, give off a pleasant fragrance when you rub them. Early American colonists took advantage of that scent, as well as the greenish white wax covering the plant's berries, to make candles. That's why bayberry is also known as candleberry and wax myrtle. Both the wax and the dried bark of bayberry roots are used medicinally.

Therapeutic Uses:
✒ Diarrhea, fever, gingivitis, hemorrhoids, hepatitis, infections, inflammation, sore throat, vaginitis.
▧ Folk uses: Chills, colds, congestion, coughing, dermatitis, diarrhea, dysentery, flu, gastritis, itching, jaundice, sores, ulcers.

Medicinal Properties:
Some research shows that bayberry contains astringent and antibacterial compounds. Myricitrin, the active antibiotic, encourages sweating, which can help break a fever. Other research suggests that large doses tend to decrease the body's potassium level, leading to higher blood pressure and both water and sodium retention. Taking too much bayberry may make you sick to your stomach or force you to vomit.

Dosage Options:
One-half to 2 grams of powdered bayberry three times a day in a tea, ⅛ to ½ teaspoon of a liquid extract three times a day, 1 teaspoon of powdered root bark daily, or ½ teaspoon of bayberry tincture daily.

Safety Rating: 1

Precautions:
In large amounts, bayberry could elevate your blood pressure or make you retain sodium or water—all because the herb tends to rid the body of potassium. If you have high blood pressure, congestive heart failure, water retention, or kidney disease, don't take bayberry without talking to a qualified herbal expert.

BEARBERRY; UVA URSI *(Arctostaphylos uva-ursi)*

What It Is:
Throughout most of the 1800s and up until 1936, bearberry was the official recommendation for urinary tract infections in the U.S. Pharmacopeia. From the Chinese to Native Americans, people used this ground-hugging woody evergreen, a close relative of cranberry and blueberry, to treat urinary problems. Its bright red berries ripen in the fall and survive throughout the winter to feed both birds and beasts, but herbal physicians have always been more interested in the plant's oval, dark green leaves.

Therapeutic Uses:
🌿🌿 Urethritis, urinary tract infections.
🌿 Coughing, cystitis, inflammation, kidney problems, prostatitis, swelling, urethral discharge, urinary problems, venereal disease.
▦ Folk uses: Bed-wetting, bronchitis, diabetes, diarrhea, dysentery, gonorrhea, kidney stones.

Medicinal Properties:
Several phytochemicals in this plant, especially arbutin, aim squarely at urinary disorders. Some of the plant substances fight bacteria and cleanse the urinary tract; others promote excretion, deter water retention, support the kidneys, and cool inflammatory reactions. The herb works as a urinary antiseptic. If your urine is extremely alkaline, it may need to be acidified. Arbutin is transformed in the body into the antiseptic hydroquinone. Some people say that the crude extract is better than isolated arbutin because of other phytochemicals present in the plant.

Dosage Options:
One to three 500-milligram capsules three times a day, 250 to 500 milligrams of a bearberry supplement standardized for 20 percent arbutin daily, 1½ to 4 grams of dried bearberry leaves in a tea three times a day, or 1 teaspoon of bearberry tincture three times a day.

Safety Rating: 1

Precautions:
The high tannin content of bearberry can contribute to nausea, stomachache, and perhaps even vomiting if you're especially sensitive. If your urine is already acidic, don't take bearberry. Do not use for more than 2 weeks without the supervision of a qualified practitioner. Do not use if you have kidney disease.

BELLADONNA *(Atropa belladonna)*

What It Is:
In Italian, *belladonna* means "fair lady." The juice of this plant, native to central and southern Europe, dilates the pupils, which in ancient Rome supposedly enhanced beauty. However, the plant's more common and more appropriate name is deadly nightshade. Its leaves, roots, and black berries are dangerous. Even in small doses, they can kill you or send you into a coma.

Therapeutic Uses:
🌿🌿 Biliary spasms, cardiac insufficiency, colic, gallbladder problems, irregular heart rhythm, liver problems, low blood pressure, neuroses, pain, stomach disease.
▦ Folk uses: Asthma, bronchial problems, colds, fever.

Medicinal Properties:
Your ophthalmologist might very well use a prescription compound derived from belladonna to dilate your pupils so that he may better examine your eyes. That action comes courtesy of a sedating phytochemical called atropine. Other compounds in the plant make belladonna a narcotic and sedative. Such anticholinergic compounds as scopolamine and hyoscyamine first stimulate and then depress the central nervous system. They reduce bodily secretions, drying up a runny nose and interfering with perspiration, and slow the movement of food through the gastrointestinal tract.

Dosage Options:
Belladonna is not a do-it-yourself medicinal herb. Consult your health care provider.

Safety Rating:
Do not use.

Precautions:
Besides making you tired and knocking you out, belladonna may have a variety of side effects, including mental confusion, constipation, cramps, delirium, dry mouth, dry skin, flushing, hallucinations, and urinary difficulties. It can also cause heart palpitations, make you thirsty, increase the pressure inside your eyes, and raise your blood pressure.

BILBERRY (*Vaccinium myrtillus*)

What It Is:
This sweet, bluish black berry went to medical school. Some of its siblings—including cranberry, blueberry, and huckleberry—studied medicine, too, but bilberry is the true doctor in the family. The berries sprout from small, wiry branches on a shrub that grows predominantly in wooded areas of northern Europe and sections of western Asia. The ripe fruit is best for therapeutic purposes, but the leaves also are used.

Therapeutic Uses:
ᕁᕁᕁ Constipation, diarrhea, vomiting.
ᕁᕁ Cardiovascular disease, diabetic retinopathy, eye problems, glaucoma, gum disease, hardening of the arteries, hemorrhoids, indigestion, macular degeneration, menstrual irregularities, nearsightedness, night blindness, retinitis, sore throat, stomach problems.
ᕁ Bruises, cataracts, diabetes, dysentery, encephalitis, gum disease, hepatitis, high cholesterol, impaired vision, indigestion, infections, inflammation, low blood sugar, pain, poor night vision, Raynaud's disease, ulcers, urinary problems, varicose veins, water retention, wounds.
▨ Folk uses: Arthritis, atherosclerosis, chest pain, dermatitis, gastric problems, gout, high blood sugar, kidney problems, urinary problems.

Medicinal Properties:
The anthocyanosides in bilberry are big-time antioxidants that provide a lot of the medicinal punch. They tend to work their magic in the capillaries, the tiny blood vessels that fill the eyes, the skin, and all other parts of the body. By ensuring good circulation and fending off free radical damage, bilberry keeps the capillaries strong and healthy—deterring bruising, ensuring good circulation to connective tissues, preserving the blood supply to the eyes, and helping to ward off heart disease. The herb also shows some anti-inflammatory, antiseptic, and astringent qualities.

Prescription Counterparts:
Before you turn to an over-the-counter diarrhea medicine, give bilberry a try. For night blindness and retinopathy, no prescription counterpart exists.

Dosage Options:
A twice-daily dosage of two 475-milligram capsules that contain at least 10 milligrams of anthocyanosides; 240 to 480 milligrams of a supplement standardized for 25 percent anthocyanosides; ½ to 2 teaspoons of a liquid extract; or 1 to 2 tablespoons of crushed bilberry fruit in a cup of boiling water daily.

Safety Rating: 3

Precautions:
If you eat handfuls of fresh bilberries, you might get diarrhea. Other than that, the fruit is thoroughly safe. Don't consume a lot of bilberry leaves.

BIRCH (*Betula*, various species)

What It Is:
A common, flowering tree throughout temperate parts of Asia, Europe, and the United States, birch has small, shiny, serrated, oval leaves. Cut a stem, and out runs a sweet juice that's long been used to make wine, beer, and vinegar. An oil made from the bark and twigs of certain birch species tastes and smells like wintergreen.

Therapeutic Uses:
🐾🐾 Bladder stones, kidney stones, urinary tract infections, water retention.
🐾 Arthritis, lung problems, cancer, cystitis, eczema, fever, gout, kidney problems, pain, rheumatism, skin problems, viruses, warts.
▦ Folk uses: Baldness, dandruff, indigestion, inflammation, psoriasis, skin cancer, stomachache, worms, wounds.

Medicinal Properties:
Birch contains salicylate, the compound that the pharmaceutical industry borrowed from nature to make aspirin. Salicylate deters the body's production of certain prostaglandins that are linked to, among other things, inflammation, fever, and pain. Betulin and betulinic acid, two phytochemicals present in birch bark, display some antiviral, anticancer, and antitumor properties.

Dosage Options:
Try tossing a handful of birch bark, 1 to 2 teaspoons of powdered bark, or 1 to 2 tablespoons of fresh chopped birch leaves into a cup or so of boiling water. Let steep for 10 minutes and drink daily. Or take a typical dosage of 1 teaspoon of birch leaf tincture several times a day. For warts, you can rub the concentrated tea directly on your skin.

Safety Rating: 2

Precautions:
None reported from normal use, although the essential oil of birch, rich in methyl salicylate, could be toxic.

BITTER MELON (*Momordica charantia*)

What It Is:
A tropical vine with yellow flowers and red-tinged green fruit, bitter melon grows commonly throughout South America, Asia, and Africa. It's also called balsam pear, as the fruit looks like an odd cross between a cucumber and a gourd. It is the same size and shape as a cucumber, but it's textured, with gourdlike bumps. It can be grown as an annual in the United States and has a long herbal history (now backed up, to some extent, by science) as a treatment for diabetes.

Therapeutic Uses:

🌿🌿 Diabetes.

🌿 HIV, infections, inflammation, psoriasis.

▦ Folk uses: Boils, leprosy, lice.

Medicinal Properties:

Several clinical trials have shown that bitter melon extract and juice lower blood sugar in people with type 1 or type 2 diabetes. In one study of people with type 2 diabetes, 15 grams of bitter melon extract reduced their after-mealtime increase in blood sugar by more than 50 percent. In another study of people with type 2 diabetes, glucose tolerance improved in 73 percent of the participants after they drank 2 ounces of fresh bitter melon juice. People with type 1 diabetes also may benefit. A polypeptide extracted from the fruit lowered blood sugar levels when injected into people with type 1 diabetes. Other substances in bitter melon fight viruses, bacteria (including diphtheria, E. coli, salmonella, and streptococcus), and inflammation and inhibit HIV.

Prescription Counterparts:

One of the phytochemicals in bitter melon, charantin, is said to be more potent than tolbutamide, an oral drug for people with type 2 diabetes. And the polypeptide extract apparently has fewer side effects than insulin. Drinking bitter melon juice or eating the fruit might enable you to reduce your dosage of diabetes medication, but don't do so on your own. Talk to your physician, tell her of your intention to try the fruit, and keep very close tabs on your blood sugar level.

Dosage Options:

One 500-milligram capsule containing 150 milligrams of 2.5 percent bitter principle extract three times a day. Other options include eating one small melon every day (you can probably find the melons at an Asian market), taking 1 teaspoon of bitter melon tincture two or three times a day, or drinking about 2 ounces of fresh bitter melon juice daily. Some experts favor the fresh juice, but be forewarned: It is quite bitter.

Safety Rating: 1

Precautions:

High dosages might cause intestinal pain or diarrhea. In one experiment involving male dogs, 1.75 milligrams per 2.2 pounds of body weight reduced sperm production.

BLACKBERRY (*Rubus*, various species)

What It Is:
This thorny vine or bramble bears a sweet fruit that makes a great-tasting jelly. Blackberry's flowers and both its immature and ripe fruit may appear on the vine at the same time. One species of blackberry was once known as goutberry, an indication of just one of its medicinal uses.

Therapeutic Uses:
☙ Diarrhea, gastritis, hemorrhage, hemorrhoids, intestinal inflammation, mouth inflammation, sore throat.
▨ Folk uses: Gout, minor cuts and wounds, tissue swelling.

Medicinal Properties:
The fruit might taste better, but blackberry's leaves, bark, and roots contain the most healing potential. The astringent tannins in the plant constrict the blood vessels.

Dosage Options:
Make a tea by putting 1 to 2 teaspoons of chopped dried blackberry leaves, powdered root, or powdered bark in a cup of boiling water; drink a cup every day. Or, typically, up to 2 teaspoons of blackberry tincture or ½ to 1 teaspoon of a liquid root extract daily.

Safety Rating: 2

Precautions:
None reported. Blackberry is safe in reasonable amounts.

BLACK COHOSH (*Cimicifuga racemosa*)

What It Is:
This perennial plant, topped by a long plume of large white flowers, grows wild throughout the Ohio River valley and the eastern deciduous forests. For medicinal purposes, you can ignore the aboveground part of the plant—its long, smooth stems; long, compound leaves; and flowery white shoots—and head straight down to its gnarly black roots. The roots give the herb its name and its medicinal reputation: The Algonquian word *cohosh* means "rough." Because its flowers and roots emit a strong odor that repels insects, the plant is also known as bugbane. The Latin *cimicifuga* means "bug repellent."

Therapeutic Uses:
☙☙ Menopause, menstrual irregularities, nervous system problems, premenstrual tension.

🐛 Childbirth, cramps, excessive menstrual bleeding, fever, high blood pressure, hot flashes, lumbago, mammary inflammation, nervousness, sciatica, tinnitus.

▦ Folk uses: Asthma, bronchial problems, bronchitis, chorea (involuntary spasms of the face and limbs), coughing, indigestion, myalgia, neuralgia, rheumatism, snakebite, sore throat, water retention, whooping cough.

Medicinal Properties:
Colonial settlers soon learned what Native Americans long knew: Black cohosh is an herbal panacea for all sorts of female-specific health problems. One of the isoflavones in the plant's roots acts physiologically like a weak estrogen, making it potentially beneficial for everything from childbirth and menstrual cramps to menopause and premenstrual tension. In one study, the plant relieved menopause-related vaginal dryness just as well as pharmaceutical estrogen. In another experiment, black cohosh matched prescription-strength hormone replacement in reducing luteinizing hormone, which increases as natural estrogen declines, bringing on typical menopausal symptoms.

Dosage Options:
One 540-milligram capsule or 40 milligrams of a standardized extract three times a day. Other options include a tea made from ½ teaspoon of powdered root in a cup of boiling water, up to ½ teaspoon of a liquid extract, ½ to 1 teaspoon of black cohosh tincture, or 1 to 3 tablespoons of the plant's fresh roots daily.

Safety Rating: 1

Precautions:
Some people report an upset stomach or other gastric complaints. Be careful if you take black cohosh for longer than 6 months. Prolonged use could cause abdominal pain, dizziness, diarrhea, headache, joint pain, nausea, uterine irritation, and vomiting. Women shouldn't take it while pregnant or nursing a newborn. Overdoses might cause premature birth, nausea, and headache.

BLACK CURRANT (Ribes nigrum)

What It Is:
This low-lying shrub, found all over Europe, is often somewhat spiny and has black, tasty fruit. The plant's leaves and buds emit a strong, distinctive odor. A tea can be made from the leaves, but the berries contain the most health-promoting potential, perhaps more than red currant and white currant. When you press the seeds, you get an oil high in a nutrient called gamma-linolenic acid (GLA), an omega-6 fat essential for the body to make a certain inflammation-fighting prostaglandin. Goats are said to like leaves of black currant; bears favor the berries.

Therapeutic Uses for Fruit:

❧ Chills, colds, diarrhea, flu.

▦ Folk uses: Coughing, hoarseness, inflammation, sore throat, stomachache.

Therapeutic Uses for Leaves:

❧ Inflammation.

▦ Folk uses: Arthritis, bladder stones, colds, colic, convulsions, coughing, diarrhea, gout, liver problems, sore throat, urinary problems, whooping cough.

Therapeutic Uses for Seed Oil:

❧ Arthritis, autoimmune disorders, eczema, heart disease, high blood pressure, inflammation, multiple sclerosis, premenstrual symptoms.

Medicinal Properties:

Black currant fruit is a decent herbal cold remedy. Compounds in the berries are astringent, fight bacteria, and help reduce inflammation and secretions. The leaves display a little anti-inflammatory action and might help fight fungal infections. The GLA in the seed oil possesses a lot of potential to help treat multiple sclerosis, eczema, and other autoimmune disorders. Black currant seed oil is a less expensive substitute for evening primrose oil, the best source of GLA.

Dosage Options:

Six hundred to 6,000 milligrams of the fruit daily, four 250-milligram capsules of black currant fruit extract twice a day, or a glass of black currant juice daily. You can also gargle with a solution of one part fruit juice and one part water. For the dried leaves, place 1 to 2 teaspoons in a cup of boiling water. Let the brew steep for 10 minutes or so, then strain. Drink a cup three or four times a day. For the seed oil, a typical daily dose is 200 to 400 milligrams standardized for 14 to 19 percent GLA; for eczema, 1,000 milligrams twice a day.

Safety Rating:

For the fruit and seed oil, **3**; for the leaves, **1**.

Precautions:

None reported for either the fruit or the seed oil. Some research suggests that you shouldn't take black currant leaves in any form if you have water retention and tissue swelling related to heart or kidney problems.

BLACK HAW *(Viburnum prunifolium)*

What It Is:

This white-flowered shrub is native to North America, and Native Americans have long taken advantage of its bark for gynecologic problems. The plant grows up to 30 feet tall on hillsides, in wooded areas, and along shores and streams from Connecticut west to Michigan and south to Florida and Texas. In the old days, it was called cramp bark, a hint as to which part of the plant contains the most therapeutic properties.

Therapeutic Uses:
🔊 Diarrhea, fever, headache, intestinal inflammation, menstrual pain and irregularities, pain.
▩ Folk uses: Asthma, childbirth, miscarriage.

Medicinal Properties:
Cramp bark was so named for a very good reason: It contains at least four phytochemicals that facilitate uterine relaxation, two of which (aesculetin and scopoletin) also work against muscle spasms. The pain-relieving salicin in the herb is closely related chemically to aspirin.

Dosage Options:
Four to 8 milliliters of a liquid bark extract daily, 2 teaspoons of dried bark in a cup of boiling water daily, 2 teaspoons of black haw tincture three times a day, or a supplement containing 1 to 2 grams of powdered bark every day.

Safety Rating: 1

Precautions:
If you have kidney stones, you might want to watch how much black haw you take, given the plant's oxalates. Some evidence suggests that black haw might aggravate tinnitus, or ringing in the ears. Other than that, there are no reported problems.

BLACK WALNUT *(Juglans nigra)*

What It Is:
This deciduous forest tree grows up to 60 feet tall throughout the eastern part of the United States. Other varieties are found in Great Britain, Greece, and parts of the Middle East. Its hard wood makes for attractive cabinets and furniture, and its hard green fruit (nuts) fall like cannonballs during the autumn months. These nuts make a great snack, but the bark, leaves, and nut husks also contain natural phytomedicine.

Therapeutic Uses:
🔊 Bedbugs, diarrhea, fungal diseases, hemorrhoids, hypoactive thyroid, ringworm, sore throat, worms, wounds, yeast.
▩ Folk uses: Bruises, colic, constipation, inflammation, toothache.

Medicinal Properties:
Black walnut's antifungal, antiseptic, astringent, and antiviral properties, due in part to a chemical called juglone, make it a good weapon against all sorts of bugs,

both those that fly around in the air and those that can inhabit your body. Most notable among the latter are the candidas that cause vaginal yeast infections. The nuts contain our second-best dietary source of the mood-relaxing, nerve-easing brain chemical serotonin. (The butternut, a close relative, is the better, albeit lesser-known, source.)

Prescription Counterparts:
In one study, fresh black walnut husks killed candida yeast better than commonly prescribed antifungal medications.

Dosage Options:
Up to 495 milligrams of black walnut husks three times a day, or 10 to 20 drops of a liquid extract, 2 to 3 teaspoons of fresh nut husks, or 1 to 1½ grams of dried husks daily.

Safety Rating: 1

Precautions:
With normal use, no side effects have been reported. However, the juglone in black walnut can cause genetic mutations, and chronic use, at least according to test tube experiments, has carcinogenic effects.

BLESSED THISTLE *(Cnicus benedictus)*

What It Is:
Whether called blessed thistle, holy thistle, or St. Benedict's thistle, the name suggests the high esteem in which this plant—with hairy stems, spiny-edged leaves, and yellow flowers—was held by medieval monks. They considered it a cure for everything from smallpox to headaches. Do not confuse blessed thistle with milk thistle (see "Milk Thistle" on page 149). They are two entirely different plants, despite what some herbalists say and the fact that they share a common name (holy thistle).

Therapeutic Uses:
🌿🌿 Dry mouth, indigestion, lack of appetite.
🌿 Arthritis, bacterial infections, bursitis, cancer, colic, diarrhea, inflammation, liver problems, mucous membrane inflammation, sores, stomach problems, water retention, wounds.
▦ Folk uses: Gangrene, heartburn, menstrual irregularities.

Medicinal Properties:
According to research on lab mice, all parts of the plant show some ability to combat tumors. The active constituent, cnicin, cools inflammation, fights bacteria, and reduces fluid retention.

Prescription Counterparts:
Some reports suggest that cnicin extract has as much anti-inflammatory power as indomethacin.

Dosage Options:
Two 360-milligram capsules of blessed thistle extract three times a day, 1½ to 3 milliliters of a liquid extract three times a day, 1½ to 2 teaspoons of chopped dried blessed thistle leaves in a cup of hot water before meals, 2 to 4 tablespoons of the fresh herb every day, or 3 to 6 grams of the dried herb daily.

Safety Rating: 2

Precautions:
Large doses, such as more than 5 grams in a cup of tea, may upset the stomach and provoke vomiting. Because of its gastric effects, you should avoid the herb if you have an ulcer. Some people might have an allergic reaction to blessed thistle.

BLOODROOT *(Sanguinaria canadensis)*

What It Is:
A spring wildflower that grows in eastern deciduous forests as far west as Kansas, bloodroot takes its name from the crimson color of its roots. Native Americans used the red juice from bloodroot for face and body paint, as well as to dye cloth.

Therapeutic Uses:
◕ Bad breath, bronchitis, coughing, croup, dysentery, fungal infections, gingivitis, nasal polyps, periodontitis, sore throat, vaginal infections.
▨ Folk uses: Arthritis, asthma, cancer, colds, fever, rheumatism.

Medicinal Properties:
The very well studied sanguinarine derived from bloodroot is an excellent antiseptic that prevents bacteria from forming plaque on teeth, deterring both tooth decay and gum disease. Research shows that it reduces plaque accumulation in only 8 days and also reduces gum bleeding. Sanguinarine possesses anti-inflammatory, antihistamine, and antimicrobial properties. In addition, the herb is an expectorant that helps induce vomiting.

Prescription Counterparts:
Dentists use products that contain sanguinarine to treat gum disease. The phytochemical also is a main ingredient in commercially available mouthwashes and toothpastes (such as Viadent). You will find sanguinarine in anticough preparations, too.

Dosage Options:

Look for sanguinarine in toothpastes, mouthwashes, and perhaps cough syrups. Brush or gargle with the product and then spit it out. Do not ingest sanguinarine in any other form (see "Precautions").

Safety Rating:

Aside from toothpastes and mouthwashes, do not use any supplemental or topical preparations of bloodroot that you might find in health food stores or herbal apothecaries. It's a dangerous herb.

Precautions:

The sanguinarine extracted from bloodroot is safe and effective in the small amounts found in commercial dental products. Forms of the whole herb are, however, taboo. According to some scientists, bloodroot can contribute to glaucoma or induce a temporary case of tunnel vision. In their raw state, the roots and root juice are escharotic—that is, they actually corrode or similarly burn and damage tissue, enough to produce a scab. That's why folk physicians once used bloodroot to treat ringworm and other external growths, as well as some skin cancers.

BLUEBERRY *(Vaccinium angustifolium; V. corymbosum)*

What It Is:

Good by the handful, as a jelly or syrup, or in muffins or pancakes, blueberry belongs to the same genus *(Vaccinium)* as bilberry, bearberry, and cranberry.

Therapeutic Uses:

~ Childbirth, colic, diarrhea, inflammation, pain, sore throat, stomach problems.

Medicinal Properties:

Blueberry contains many of the same anthocyanosides as bilberry, though in smaller amounts. Although it promotes overall good health, if you're looking for a bigger herbal wallop against poor night vision, eye health, or capillary strength, stick with bilberry—or eat twice as many blueberries.

Dosage Options:

Three tablespoons of dried blueberry daily or 1 to 2 tablespoons of chopped dried blueberry leaves steeped in a cup of boiling water up to six times a day.

Safety Rating: 3

This rating applies to the fruit. The leaves generally are not ingested.

Precautions:

None reported.

BLUE COHOSH *(Caulophyllum thalictroides)*

What It Is:
Despite the same surname, blue cohosh is not closely related to black cohosh, although both have traditionally been used for gynecologic disorders. *Cohosh* is an Algonquian word meaning "rough." The description refers to the plant's roots. As you might expect, blue cohosh, which grows wild from the Appalachians west to the Mississippi River, has a bluish stem.

Therapeutic Uses:
 Arthritis, worms.
 Folk uses: Absence of menstruation, anxiety, asthma, colic, coughing, epilepsy, fever, high blood pressure, induction of labor, intestinal problems, lung problems, menstrual pain and irregularities, miscarriage, pain, rheumatism, senility, urinary tract infections, yeast infections.

Medicinal Properties:
Native Americans called it papoose root, probably because of the phytochemical caulosaponin, which is capable of triggering powerful contractions of the uterus (hence its folk use to induce childbirth and encourage menstruation). Other research suggests that the plant possesses some anti-inflammatory, antiseptic, antispasmodic, and antirheumatic properties. Its active phytochemicals also might interfere with impregnation, raise blood pressure, and speed intestinal motility.

Prescription Counterparts:
Blue cohosh probably is no more dangerous than its pharmaceutical rival, the labor-inducing oxytocin (Pitocin). This prescription medication can cause heart disease, not to mention death of the mother and fetus.

Dosage Options:
Not for self-medication (see "Precautions"). Consult a qualified physician.

Safety Rating: 1

Precautions:
This is not an herb to take on your own. The berries are poisonous, the roots irritate mucous membranes, and the leaves and stem irritate the skin. Preparations could affect a woman's menstrual cycle and might change nature's own schedule for labor. Consult with a qualified naturopathic physician.

BOLDO *(Peumus boldus)*

What It Is:

An evergreen tree indigenous to Chile and reportedly established in the mountains of some Mediterranean countries, boldo has somewhat thick, brittle, oval leaves. Chileans are said to eat the plant's yellow green fruit, strip its bark for use in tanning, and make charcoal from its wood. The plant gives off a rather unusual scent of wormseed or epasote *(Chenopodium ambrosioides)*. Its crushed leaves are particularly malodorous.

Therapeutic Uses:

🍂🍂 Indigestion, intestinal problems, liver dysfunction, loss of appetite, muscle tension, stomach disease.

🍂 Autoimmune disorders, cancer, cramps, cystitis, gallstones, gonorrhea, hardening of the arteries, inflammation, stomachache, worms.

▦ Folk uses: Gout, obesity, rheumatism.

Medicinal Properties:

In the right amounts, active constituents in boldo leaves stimulate the entire gastrointestinal tract, making them useful for a range of stomach, intestinal, and liver complaints. Boldo's mild anti-inflammatory and antiseptic actions might come into play against urinary tract infections.

Dosage Options:

One to 2 teaspoons of dried boldo leaves in a cup of boiling water daily, up to ⅛ teaspoon of a liquid extract daily, or ⅛ to ½ teaspoon of boldo tincture three times a day.

Safety Rating: 1

Precautions:

Some of the compounds in the plant can be toxic, so don't take too much and don't take it for too long; consult a qualified physician. Avoid if you have a kidney problem, gallstones, or a serious liver problem. One alkaloid in the tree's leaves, boldine, can paralyze nerves when injected under the skin. Ingestion of high dosages can cause excitement, cramps, convulsions, and increased urination.

BONESET *(Eupatorium perfoliatum)*

What It Is:
You won't be fixing fractures or warding off osteoporosis with this perennial herb. The name is derived from the plant's traditional use to treat breakbone fever, which is now known as dengue, a viral infection that causes such intense muscle pain that sufferers think their bones will break. Boneset, whose family members include daisies, dandelion, and marigolds, grows naturally in prairies and along shores and swamps throughout much of North America. The plant features long, pointy leaves and flat-topped clusters of small whitish flowers. The herb is best used for fending off fevers and counteracting colds.

Therapeutic Uses:
Arthritis, bronchitis, cancer, colds, dengue, dermatitis, flu, gout, inflammation, pleurisy, pneumonia, sore throat, tumors, urethritis.

Folk uses: Constipation, fever, indigestion, loss of appetite, malaria, muscle pain, typhoid.

Medicinal Properties:
The phytochemicals in boneset help rev up the immune system's white blood cells against viruses and other microorganisms, explaining its longtime use against colds and flu. Aside from its anti-inflammatory action, it encourages the body to perspire, thus two of its other common names, sweat plant and feverwort. Native Americans and colonial settlers used it to treat a variety of fever-causing afflictions.

Prescription Counterparts:
In the old days, boneset was a top-notch drug. Only the advent of aspirin displaced it as the most popular choice for colds and fevers.

Dosage Options:
One to 2 teaspoons of chopped dried boneset leaves in a cup of boiling water, ¼ to ½ teaspoon of a liquid extract, or ¼ to 1 teaspoon of boneset tincture three times a day. You might want to add some honey or sugar to the tea, as the plant is quite bitter.

Safety Rating: 1

Precautions:
Consumption of large amounts can induce nausea, vomiting, and diarrhea. Some of the active constituents might cause skin reactions. If you're allergic to chamomile, feverfew, or ragwort, you might be allergic to boneset.

BORAGE *(Borago officinalis)*

What It Is:
You might find borage's blue star-shaped flowers in that potpourri you have sitting on the shelf in your bathroom. You also may find it growing wild throughout the eastern United States, where it was introduced from Europe. Fresh leaves have a crisp, cucumber-like scent and a cooling effect that complements salads, syrups, jams, teas, and other drinks. In days of old when knights were bold, as the saying grows cold, jousters believed that borage brought them courage.

Therapeutic Uses:
◣ Arthritis, colds, dermatitis, diarrhea, heart problems, inflammation, menopause, premenstrual tension, stress.

▣ Folk uses: Bronchial problems, corns, coughing, depression, fever, jaundice, kidney stones, phlebitis, sore throat, wounds.

Medicinal Properties:
Like evening primrose and black currant seeds (see "Evening Primrose" on page 96 and "Black Currant" on page 41), borage seeds are another source of gamma-linolenic acid (GLA), the omega-6 fatty acid that the body uses to make an inflammation-fighting, autoimmune-boosting prostaglandin. Some research conducted during cardiac stress tests indicates that borage oil lowers systolic blood pressure and heart rate.

Dosage Options:
Three hundred milligrams of a standardized extract containing 24 percent GLA daily, ½ to 1 teaspoon of a liquid leaf extract daily, ¼ to 1 teaspoon of borage tincture three times a day, or 2 teaspoons of the dried herb in a cup of boiling water three times a day.

Safety Rating: 1

Precautions:
Several herbalists caution against prolonged or excessive use of products containing borage. The pyrrolizidine alkaloids (PAs) in the plant are known to be toxic and possibly carcinogenic. (For more information on PAs, see "Coltsfoot" on page 81.) Borage oil, however, contains very little, if any, of these compounds.

BOSWELLIA *(Boswellia commiphora; B. serrata)*

What It Is:
The next time Christmas rolls around, don't think frankincense and myrrh; think boswellia. Since the biblical birth of Christ, frankincense, myrrh, boswellia, and other resin-releasing desert shrubs of the ancient Holy Land have been confused with one another. Today the wisest of botanists and chemists can't differentiate among the various members of the Burseraceae family (especially in the *Boswellia* and *Commiphora* genera), all now thought to be myrrh, even when the plants are in full bloom. One botanical name of frankincense is *B. thurifera;* one botanical name of myrrh is *B. commiphora.* We'll probably never know precisely what resinous substances the three wise men toted across the desert to present to the Christ child (all of these plants bleed a sticky resin that was probably burned as incense), but someday we might learn the full medicinal secrets of these fragrant herbs.

Therapeutic Uses:
❧ Arthritis, bursitis, colitis, Crohn's disease, hepatitis, inflammation, ringworm.
▒ Folk uses: Boils, diarrhea, wrinkles.

Medicinal Properties:
Boswellia's two major phytochemicals, boswellin and boswellic acid, possess some anti-arthritic, anti-inflammatory, and diuretic properties. We don't know much more because we Westerners haven't been around this Johnny-come-lately long enough to uncover its health potential.

Dosage Options:
Four hundred milligrams of a supplement standardized for 37.5 percent boswellic acid three times a day. Depending on the brand, you might find supplements of whole boswellia or extracts of either of its main active ingredients.

Safety Rating: 2

Precautions:
Side effects are rare, but particularly sensitive people might experience diarrhea, an upset stomach, or a skin rash.

BROMELAIN (Bromeliaceae, from *Ananas comosus*)

See "Pineapple" on page 173.

BROOM *(Cytisus scoparius; Sarothamnus scoparius)*

What It Is:

Do not confuse broom, also called Scotch broom, with butcher's broom (see "Butcher's Broom" on page 57). Native to Europe but now found in South America and all over North America, broom, with its small, bright yellow leaves, belongs to the pea family and has a long history as an herbal medicine. At one time, the plant's tender green tops were used as a flavoring agent in beer. Its most common use, however, was custodial: The first part of one of the botanical names, *Sarothamnus*, is derived from a Greek verb meaning "to sweep." The last part of this botanical name, *scoparius*, is derived from the Latin word meaning "besom," a broom made out of twigs. In short, the flexible, durable sticks and stems of the plant's branches make excellent brooms.

Therapeutic Uses:

🍂🍂 Circulatory problems, heart disease.
🍂 Irregular heart rhythm, low blood pressure.
▦ Folk uses: Abscesses, childbirth, gallstones, gout, hemophilia, jaundice, kidney stones, liver problems, lung problems, muscle pain, palpitations, rapid heart rate, rheumatism, sciatica, snakebite, tumors, water retention.

Medicinal Properties:

Qualified herbalists have long used this potent plant to encourage excretion, improve poor circulation, stabilize irregular heart rhythm, and treat other heart problems. The primary phytochemical in broom, sparteine, is a cardiac depressant powerful enough, in sulfate form, to cause respiratory arrest, high blood pressure, and uterine contractions. Dosages of about 30 grams (containing more than 300 milligrams of sparteine) may also cause dizziness, a feeling of weakness in the legs, headache, sleepiness, and a tingling sensation in the hands and feet. The tyramine in broom reportedly raises blood pressure and constricts the veins.

Prescription Counterparts:

Sparteine is often compared to the heart-depressing prescription drug quinidine (Quinaglute). In fact, in Germany physicians consider broom on a par with quinidine for irregular heart rhythm. Quinidine has its perils, but so does broom. Only an experienced, herb-savvy physician can decide which, if either, is better for you.

Dosage Options:

Not for self-medication (see "Precautions").

Safety Rating:

Do not use on your own. Take only under the supervision of a knowledgeable practitioner.

Precautions:
While Germany's Commission E has okayed the use of broom, it is too powerful for self-medicating purposes. It's more likely to cause, rather than cure, high blood pressure, yet the widely cited PDR for Herbal Medicines lists it as a good natural remedy for hypertension. Sparteine triggers strong uterine contractions and slows cardiac function. Small doses might stimulate the heart, but larger doses definitely will depress it. Large amounts also will induce vomiting, impair vision, and cause sweating. The FDA labels it a poisonous herb.

BUCHU *(Barosma betulina; Agathosma betulina)*

What It Is:
We in the industrialized world have long relied on pharmaceuticals to encourage urinary excretion and deter water retention. In Namibia and South Africa, however, traditional medicine has relied even longer on this shrubby member of the orange and lemon family for its diuretic effect. The plant produces a brown fruit from its small white flowers, but its leaves, which smell like peppermint, are considered the most medicinally active part.

Therapeutic Uses:
🍂 Cystitis, prostatitis, urethral infections, water retention.
▨ Folk uses: Bruises, heart disease, high blood pressure, inflammation, kidney stones, premenstrual tension, urinary tract infections, venereal disease.

Medicinal Properties:
The diosphenol in buchu helps kill bacteria, so I tend to endorse this herbal medicine for the urinary complaints for which it's long been used.

Prescription Counterparts:
If you use certain over-the-counter premenstrual diuretics (such as Fluidex or Odrinil) to reduce water retention, you're already taking buchu. Both products contain the herb as an active ingredient. If a doctor has prescribed a pharmaceutical diuretic for your high blood pressure, talk to an herb-friendly physician to see whether this natural alternative might help reduce your dependence on the drug.

Dosage Options:
One teaspoon of dried leaves in a cup of boiling water several times a day, 10 to 30 drops of a liquid buchu extract in a glass of water or juice daily, or ½ to 1 teaspoon of a liquid leaf extract daily.

Safety Rating: 2

Precautions:
Although the FDA deems buchu safe, if you have kidney disease, take the herb cautiously. The pulegone and diosphenol might irritate your liver. Any diuretic, natural

or synthetic, tends to reduce the body's potassium level, so make sure to eat more bananas and other potassium-rich foods. There is a slight chance that herbal extracts might cause diarrhea or stomach upset. If so, don't take as much.

BUCKWHEAT *(Fagopyrum esculentum)*

What It Is:
A sprawling herb with a knotty, hollow stem and whitish flowers, buckwheat is native to northern and central Asia but is now commonly cultivated in North America. Buckwheat flour comes from the plant's dark brown, triangular fruit, which most people would call a nut. The fruit resembles the three-sided beechnut (Fagus), from which buckwheat's scientific name is derived.

Therapeutic Uses:
Chronic venous insufficiency, colon cancer, tissue swelling, varicose veins, water retention.

Folk use: Hardening of the arteries.

Medicinal Properties:
Buckwheat's high content of the bioflavonoid rutin makes it an excellent choice for anyone concerned about varicose veins or hardening of the arteries. Rutin bucks up the strength of the capillaries. Weak veins and capillaries allow blood and fluid to back up and leak into nearby tissues. Depending on where the weakness is, you might get varicose veins or hemorrhoids.

Dosage Options:
You probably won't find buckwheat in supplement form anywhere, but it's sound "food farmacy." One-half cup of buckwheat flour might contain about 6,000 milligrams of rutin. Just cook up a stack of buckwheat pancakes and drizzle some blueberry syrup on top. Blueberry contains its own capillary-strengthening phytochemical, making it a smart (and tasty) complement. Or perhaps you might find some buckwheat honey. In some parts of the United States and elsewhere, the plant is grown as bee food.

Safety Rating: 3

Precautions:
Virtually none—for most of us. Just as a few individuals are highly allergic to peanuts, a few people might experience a rare but very lethal anaphylactic reaction to buckwheat.

BUGLE (*Lycopus europaeus; L. virginicus*)

What It Is:
This low, creeping perennial, with its small, blue purple or white flowers, carpets fields, roadsides, and lawns from Newfoundland to Ohio. The white corkscrew-shaped root is edible, and the entire plant is used in herbal medicine.

Therapeutic Uses:
🕭🕭 Breast pain, hyperthyroidism (Graves' disease), hypothyroidism, insomnia, nervousness, premenstrual tension.
🕭 Coughing.
▦ Folk uses: Anxiety, cardiopathy, diabetes, lung problems, palpitations.

Medicinal Properties:
If the research is accurate, bugle helps your thyroid. Apparently, it doesn't matter whether that gland in your neck secretes too much or too little of its hormones. Bugle seems to stabilize everything, revving up production if the thyroid produces too little and curtailing production and deterring the metabolism of iodine, the mineral on which the gland relies, if it's in overdrive. People with hyperthyroidism typically are restless, irritable, and frequently tired. Other symptoms include excessive sweating, bulging eyes, a fast pulse, and drastic weight loss.

Prescription Counterparts:
For an overactive thyroid, mainstream medicine often prefers to destroy the gland with radiation, then prescribe synthetic thyroid replacement, on which you become dependent for the rest of your life. Consider talking to an herb-savvy physician about using bugle before exposing your neck to tissue-killing radiation.

Dosage Options:
Under a doctor's supervision only, take 0.2 to 2 grams of the raw herb or ⅛ to ½ teaspoon of a liquid extract daily. Bugle leaves contain more active ingredients than bugle roots. Alcohol-extracted root tinctures are best. In Europe, bugle often is combined with lemon balm (see "Lemon Balm" on page 139) to treat the early stages of Graves' disease.

Safety Rating: 2

Precautions:
Despite the safety of the herb, if you have a thyroid problem you should be under a doctor's supervision. Don't take bugle if you're already taking prescription thyroid supplements. If you start to take the herb regularly, don't stop suddenly; decrease your dosage gradually. Extracts will reduce the body's secretion of prolactin, one of the hormones necessary to manufacture breast milk. Extracts also may deter the production of other gonadotropic hormones, including estrogen and testosterone.

BURDOCK *(Arctium lappa)*

What It Is:

A biennial weed from the aster family that may grow up to 6 to 8 feet tall, burdock came from Europe and now can be found in fields and along roads throughout North America as far north as Michigan and Quebec; as far south as Pennsylvania, Illinois, and even Alabama; and as far west as California. It features large leaves, some with heartlike notches at the bottom, and purplish flowers that precede the small burs that harden as they ripen. The plant's roots are considered vegetables in Japan, as common as carrots in the United States. Young burdock leaf stalks are a good addition to soups but too bitter for salads.

Therapeutic Uses:

➴ Bladder stones, boils, high blood sugar, lymphoma, psoriasis, tumors.

▩ Folk uses: Acne, anorexia, arthritis, backache, bruises, burns, canker sores, colds, constipation, cystitis, dermatitis, dizziness, eczema, flu, gout, hair loss, indigestion, liver problems, high blood sugar, hives, kidney stones and other problems, measles, pain, scarlet fever, sciatica, seborrhea, smallpox, sores, stomach problems, syphilis, ulcers, urinary tract infections, warts, wounds.

Medicinal Properties:

Fresh burdock roots contain phytochemicals called polyacetylenes, which can destroy certain bacteria and fungi, perhaps explaining the traditional use of this herb as a treatment for ringworm, urinary tract infections, and other bacterial onslaughts. One study demonstrated that an extract reduced blood sugar and improved carbohydrate tolerance in lab rats. Certain lignans might help ward off cancer.

Dosage Options:

You can eat burdock roots and leaves as cooked vegetables, or you can munch on the cooked stalks as you would celery. Other options include 1,410 milligrams of burdock capsules three times a day, ½ to 2 teaspoons of a liquid root extract daily, ⅛ to ½ teaspoon of a liquid seed extract daily, a tea made from 1¼ teaspoons of chopped or powdered burdock root daily, or 2 teaspoons to 1 tablespoon of a root tincture three times a day. For seborrhea, massage burdock root oil into your scalp.

Safety Rating: 3

Precautions:

Virtually none. Some slight evidence suggests that poultices made from burdock roots might cause contact dermatitis in a few sensitive people.

BURNET *(Sanguisorba officinalis)*

What It Is:
Also called salad burnet and greater burnet, the plant, introduced from Europe, now grows naturally in various parts of the eastern, central, and western United States. Its serrated, ovate leaves taste a little like cucumber and can be used in salads.

Therapeutic Uses:
🗫🗫 Dermatitis, dysentery, eczema.
🗫 Burns, gum disease, hemorrhoids, ulcerative colitis, uterine bleeding.
▨ Folk uses: Boils, diarrhea, hemorrhage, hot flashes, phlebitis, varicose veins, wounds.

Medicinal Properties:
Burnet's botanical first name is a tip-off to its therapeutic potential. The Latin word *sanguisorba* means "blood absorber." Phytochemicals in burnet have antihemorrhagic, astringent, and styptic qualities, making it an herbal choice against ulcerative colitis, diarrhea, and uterine bleeding. It's mildly antimicrobial, fights tissue swelling, and deters wound weeping—all reasons for its use on burns.

Dosage Options:
Two to 6 grams of dried burnet tops in a cup of boiling water, ½ to 1 teaspoon of a liquid tops extract, or ½ to 2 teaspoons of burnet tincture three times a day. If you can find burnet leaves, try them in a salad.

Safety Rating: 2

Precautions:
None reported.

BUTCHER'S BROOM *(Ruscus aculeatus)*

What It Is:
This low, woody, perennial evergreen, close to the lily family, grows throughout Europe, the northern part of Africa, and western Asia, but it's hardy enough to survive just about anywhere. From its stems sprout numerous short branches and even more stiff leaves—perfect material to be gathered together in broomlike fashion, hence the plant's name. The greenish white flowers give way to scarlet berries that are the size of small cherries. The whole herb, but particularly its rhizome, contains herbal medicine.

Therapeutic Uses:
🌿🌿 Chronic venous insufficiency, hemorrhoids, inflammation.
🌿 Arthritis, blood clotting, cramps, itching, pain, phlebitis, swelling, varicose veins.
▦ Folk uses: Atherosclerosis, fractures.

Medicinal Properties:
Butcher's broom deserves its long-standing reputation for treating hemorrhoids, varicose veins, and other vein-related problems. The two active ingredients in its rhizome, ruscogenin and neoruscogenin, constrict veins, strengthen the walls of blood vessels, and reduce inflammation. One clinical trial tested the herb on 40 people with pain, swelling, itching, and cramps in their legs—all signs of chronic venous insufficiency. Symptoms improved markedly for those who took an extract standardized for ruscogenin, and no one complained of any side effects.

Dosage Options:
A standardized extract containing 50 to 100 milligrams of ruscogenin, a raw extract providing 7 to 11 milligrams of ruscogenin or ruscogenin and neoruscogenin, 1 to 2 tablespoons of fresh butcher's broom roots, or 5 teaspoons of dried roots in a cup of boiling water daily.

Safety Rating: 2

Precautions:
None reported, except for a rare case of nausea or other gastric complaints.

CALENDULA *(Calendula officinalis)*

What It Is:
With those bright, yellow orange flowers, you might mistake calendula for any other marigold. (It is, in fact, also known as pot marigold.) But calendula is actually an entirely different plant. It's native to northern Africa and the south-central portion of Europe, but it can be grown elsewhere, including indoors. If you can't visually distinguish calendula from marigold, you'll probably be more successful using

your nose: Regular garden marigolds (*Tagetes* species) give off a strong, unpleasant aroma (although some people like it); calendula is comparatively milder.

Therapeutic Uses:

❧❧ Burns, inflammation, mucositis, pharyngitis, sores, sore throat, wounds.

❧ Bunions, dermatitis, enlarged lymph glands, indigestion, infections, otitis (ear inflammation), spasms, tumors, water retention.

▣ Folk uses: Abrasions, acne, bee stings, breast pain, cancer, convulsions, coughing, cramps, dry eyes, eczema, fever, frostbite, gas, gastritis, hemorrhoids, jaundice and other liver problems, menstrual irregularities, phlebitis, skin problems, sore throat, strep throat, sunburn, thrombophlebitis, toothache, varicose veins, water retention, worms.

Medicinal Properties:

The phytochemicals in calendula oppose fungi, bacteria, viruses, and inflammation. They also excite white blood cells in the immune system to fight microbial invaders with a little more vigor. For these reasons and others, calendula has been a good treatment for skin problems of all kinds, particularly cuts, scrapes, bruises, and minor wounds.

Dosage Options:

For a sore throat or indigestion, drink calendula tea or use it to gargle; for physical injuries, apply the tea right to your skin. Dosage possibilities include 1 to 4 grams of calendula flowers in a cup of boiling water, ⅛ to ¼ teaspoon of a liquid flower extract, or 5 to 40 drops of calendula tincture three times a day. To apply topically, steep 1 teaspoon of dried petals in a cup of boiling water for 10 minutes or so. Dip a cloth in the liquid and apply as a compress. Or look for a calendula-containing cream or ointment in a health food store.

Safety Rating: 3

Precautions:

Aside from one vague report out of Russia in which someone went into anaphylactic shock after gargling with a calendula concoction, no major side effects or warnings are known. If you're allergic to ragweed, though, you might be allergic to calendula.

CAMPHOR *(Cinnamomum camphora)*

What It Is:

The aromatic wood and essential oil of this towering tree native to eastern Asia were extremely popular in nineteenth-century America and Europe. The rugged wood is a natural moth and insect repellent, while the oil from the leaves, roots, and branches was thought to relieve colds and all sorts of aches, pains, and other physical complaints. As a treatment, people once commonly hung tiny bags of camphor crystals around their necks or inhaled the oil's vapors.

Therapeutic Uses:
✎ Bacterial infections, bronchitis, congestion, coughing, heart disease, irregular heart rhythm, itching, muscle pain, nervousness.

▥ Folk uses: Arthritis, burns, chilblains, colds, cold sores, diarrhea, hemorrhoids, herpes.

Medicinal Properties:
The derivative of the camphor tree, known chemically as 2-bornanone and popularly as camphor, does indeed fight infections, redden the skin, ease muscle pain, and act as a counterirritant.

Prescription Counterparts:
Some over-the-counter back salves and cold rubs still contain camphor (check the labels).

Dosage Options:
If you use an over-the-counter product that contains camphor, follow the label directions to the letter. Use it only externally and only for a brief time. Do not apply for a prolonged period.

Safety Rating:
Do not use. If you use a camphor-containing product, do not ingest it.

Precautions:
Keep camphor away from children. The fumes are toxic, particularly if camphor ointment is applied to kids' faces. Adults would be wise to keep it away from their noses, too. No one should be exposed to this herbal extract in any form on a long-term basis. Some people who apply camphor salves may contract eczema. Don't rub camphor compounds on burned or broken skin.

CARAWAY 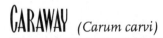 *(Carum carvi)*

What It Is:
If you've ever eaten a piece of rye bread, you've no doubt eaten caraway. The fruit of this biennial member of the carrot family looks like a seed (and is so called) and has long been used in baking. The plant, with its tiny white or red-tinged flower clusters, is native to Africa and Eurasia but now grows wild over much of North America.

Therapeutic Uses:
◐◐ Bronchitis, colds, coughing, fever, gallbladder problems, lack of appetite, sore throat.
◐ Anemia, bacterial infections, colic, cramps, gas, indigestion, infections, liver problems, muscle spasms, stomach problems, yeast infections.
▦ Folk uses: Breast milk deficiency, heart disease, incontinence, menstrual pain and irregularities, nausea, nervousness.

Medicinal Properties:
Caraway contains mild antihistamines, antimicrobial compounds (particularly against bacterial and candida infections), and muscle relaxants that help check spasms. It also cuts down on intestinal gas—all reasons the seeds have been considered good digestive aids since ancient Egyptian times.

Dosage Options:
One to 2 teaspoons of crushed caraway seeds in a cup of boiling water up to four times a day, ½ to 1 teaspoon of caraway tincture three times a day, or ¾ to 1 teaspoon of a liquid extract three or four times a day. For a little "food farmacy," munch on a teaspoon of whole caraway seeds three or four times a day. Or sprinkle them on a loaf of home-baked bread or a salad.

Safety Rating: 2

Precautions:
If you have a kidney problem, you might want to stay away from caraway. Otherwise, you should be fine.

CARDAMOM *(Elettaria cardamomum)*

What It Is:
The large perennial herb that gives us cardamom seeds grows chiefly in southern India, although it's now cultivated widely as a money crop elsewhere, especially in Guatemala and Costa Rica. Inside the somewhat tiny, triangular, pale yellow or gray fruit are two rows of seeds from which we obtain this aromatic spice. For centuries, people in Arab countries have used cardamom as an aphrodisiac, probably because it tends to stimulate the central nervous system.

Therapeutic Uses:
◐◐ Bronchitis, colds, fever, gallbladder problems, indigestion, infections, lack of appetite, liver problems, mouth inflammation, sore throat.
◐ Bad breath, colic, cramps, fatigue, gas, stomachache.
▦ Folk uses: Asthma, urinary problems.

Medicinal Properties:
Cardamom is perhaps the best source of a phytochemical called cineole, a strong antiseptic that kills the bacteria responsible for bad breath. Cineole also helps break up chest congestion and gives the entire central nervous system a boost.

Dosage Options:
Fifteen crushed seeds in a cup of hot water up to five times a day, ½ to 2 grams of cardamom powder daily, or ½ to 1 teaspoon of cardamom tincture or a liquid extract daily.

Safety Rating: 2

Precautions:
None reported, although people with gallstones should talk to a phytochemical physician before taking the herb.

CAROB (Ceratonia siliqua)

What It Is:
This well-known, stimulant-free chocolate substitute used to be called St. John's bread and locust bean. It grows primarily in the Mediterranean areas of southern Europe, Africa, and Asia. Carob trees may grow up to 30 feet tall, and their wood has a pinkish tint. The chocolate alternative comes from the pulp inside pods that grow 6 to 12 inches long from the tree's small red flowers.

Therapeutic Uses:
๏๏ Bacterial infections, diarrhea, indigestion.
๏ Heartburn.

Medicinal Properties:
Carob's usefulness was validated in a study of 41 babies with bacterial or viral diarrhea. The infants given carob recovered within 2 days; those treated with conventional medicine took almost twice as long to get better. The carob kids also stopped vomiting and regained normal temperatures and body weights quicker. Why did the chocolate substitute work? Its tannins inhibit bacteria and bind with certain toxins, inactivating them and allowing them to pass through the body. Curiously, carob is also high in fiber, which encourages bowel movements. Although that seems somewhat contradictory for a diarrhea treatment, it perhaps explains carob's effectiveness against heartburn: The fiber makes stomach contents more viscous, thus deterring the backflow of acid into the throat.

Dosage Options:
Adults can take 15 to 20 grams of carob a day, mixed with something equally tasty, such as applesauce. The infant diarrhea study used 1½ grams of carob pod powder

for every 2.2 pounds of body weight. The powder was mixed in either milk or a fluid that helped prevent dehydration.

Safety Rating: 3

Precautions:
Because of the threat of dehydration, an infant with diarrhea should be under the watchful care of a pediatrician. Don't try the carob cure on your own.

CASCARA SAGRADA *(Rhamnus purshiana)*

What It Is:
Even botanists and herbalists have a tough time distinguishing among the different species of this berry-bearing tree, so physicians and chemists don't have a chance. All the variants belong to the buckthorn family. Alder buckthorn *(Frangula alnus)* and common buckthorn *(Rhamnus cathartica)* grow in Europe; cascara sagrada grows mostly in the Pacific Northwest, from the northern part of California north to British Columbia, but it's also been planted as far east as Maryland. All have essentially one therapeutic use: as a very strong laxative.

Cascara sagrada bark is the preferred plant medicine. Some experts say that it's milder than its buckthorn relatives and safer to use. Drying the bark and allowing it to age for a year or more also lessens its powerful purgative effect. The name, by the way, means "sacred bark"—an indication of the extent to which constipation plagued early Spanish explorers in America and a testament to the effectiveness of the natural remedy.

Therapeutic Uses:
🌿🌿 Constipation
🌿 Cancer, chickenpox, flu, gas, hemorrhoids, herpes, indigestion, leukemia, ringworm, shingles.
▦ Folk uses: Arthritis, gallstones, jaundice, liver problems, sunburn prevention.

Medicinal Properties:
Thank chemicals called anthraquinones for cascara sagrada's purgative effect. A chemical reaction with bacteria in your gut changes the anthraquinones into substances that compel your intestines to contract, thus stimulating a bowel movement.

Prescription Counterparts:
So good is cascara sagrada that it's a primary active ingredient in many commercial laxatives found at health food stores.

Dosage Options:
About 10 drops of a standardized cascara sagrada extract, 1 to 3 grams of dried bark, 1 to 2½ grams of powdered bark, or ½ to 1 teaspoon of a liquid bark extract daily.

Safety Rating: 1

Precautions:
Don't rely on cascara sagrada for any length of time; consult a qualified physician. If you do, your intestines may come to depend on it for bowel movements, and you'll end up being constipated again. And certainly don't use the fresh bark, with its fully active anthraquinones, which can induce vomiting and bloody diarrhea. Other varieties of buckthorn may work even more quickly and more dramatically. Don't use cascara sagrada if you have a bad appendix, colitis, Crohn's disease, hemorrhoids, irritable bowel syndrome, a kidney problem, or any abdominal pain of unknown origin. Chronic use may increase the potency of certain heart medications and lead to a potassium deficiency. Taking too much may provoke the purge from both ends: diarrhea and vomiting. Children younger than age 12 shouldn't take it at all.

CASSIA *(Cinnamomum aromaticum)*

See "Cinnamon and Cassia" on page 111.

CATNIP *(Nepeta cataria)*

What It Is:
When you take a whiff of catnip, you'll be reminded of mint and lemon. When your cat takes a whiff, he might run around in herbal ecstasy. (Don't worry if your kitty doesn't respond; not all cats are turned on by the plant.) Catnip's green leaves, covered with a grayish down, and lavender flowers have no inebriating effect on people. If anything, the plant, which is native to Europe and now grows wild all over North America, acts the opposite way. Most of our feline friends are attracted to its oils, which nature intended to fend off bugs. The more a cat rubs against the herb, the more oil is exuded—and the more kitty goes crazy.

Therapeutic Uses:
🐾 Cataracts, cramps, glaucoma, insomnia.
▓ Folk uses: Bronchitis, colds, colic, corns, coughing, diarrhea, fever, gas, menstrual irregularities, respiratory problems, stomachache, tissue swelling.

Medicinal Properties:
Like many other members of the mint family (such as rosemary), catnip leaves contain considerable quantities of vitamins C and E, both excellent antioxidants. Flavonoids in Tabby's favorite phytochemical reserve also contribute to the plant's antioxidant might. The primary phytochemicals, nepetalactone isomers, are mild sedatives, somewhat like the active ingredients in valerian. They also quell spasms and help stimulate menstruation. The aldose reductase inhibitors might help treat cataracts.

Dosage Options:
Two teaspoons of the dried herb in a cup of hot water up to three times a day, ½ to 4 grams of the dried herb every day, or 1 teaspoon of catnip tincture three times a day. For your kitty, sew up a handful of the herb in an old sock.

Safety Rating: 2

Precautions:
In reasonable amounts, none reported, except for the usual warnings about use by pregnant women.

CAT'S CLAW *(Uncaria tomentosa)*

What It Is:
The stem and root of this woody vine, a member of the madder family, are harvested in Brazil, Peru, and other parts of the Amazon region, where it's called *uña de gato*. Only relatively recently have herbal enthusiasts in the United States taken notice of this plant, which apparently eases a variety of inflammatory and intestinal complaints. It may even figure into tomorrow's treatments for immune system problems such as HIV and cancer.

Therapeutic Uses:
☙ Allergies, arthritis, cancer, gout, hemorrhoids, HIV, immune system problems, inflammation, melanoma, prostatitis, swelling.
▦ Folk uses: Asthma, gastritis, indigestion, intestinal problems, ulcers, yeast infections.

Medicinal Properties:
Cat's claw contains a cornucopia of phytomedicinal substances. Its quinovic acid glycosides cool inflammation throughout the body. Immune system enhancement comes courtesy of the oxyindole alkaloids and proanthocyanidins, among other phytochemicals. German, Italian, and Austrian research conducted as far back as the 1970s demonstrates that compounds in cat's claw inhibit tumor growth in lab animals and petri dishes. Other European experiments have found definite

immune-strengthening effects. Still other research shows that the plant fights bacteria and viruses and reduces tissue swelling.

Prescription Counterparts:
In Austria and Germany, cat's claw preparations are bona fide, prescription-only medications. The quinovic acid glycosides, according to some reports, may shrink swelling better than the much-hyped, often-prescribed nonsteroidal anti-inflammatory drug (NSAID) indomethacin. Those phytochemicals probably won't ease an attack of gout as well as indomethacin, but they might help if you consume a sufficiently large amount.

Dosage Options:
Twenty to 60 milligrams of a standardized extract every day or one or two 500-milligram capsules of cat's claw bark three times a day. Root preparations may be up to four times stronger than preparations made from the bark.

Safety Rating: 2

Precautions:
Herbal preparations readily available over the counter in the United States are probably as safe as coffee. In Austria and Germany, though, standardized extracts are not permitted to be used along with therapies such as insulin and certain hormones. Nor may hemophiliacs receiving fresh blood plasma use the herb. Despite the favorable effects on the immune system, some overcautious authorities warn against the use of cat's claw for immune system problems such as HIV and multiple sclerosis.

CAYENNE (*Capsicum*, various species)

What It Is:
Whether you're eating Mexican, Chinese, or any cuisine in between, if the food sparks a fire in your mouth, you probably can thank a substance called capsaicin. The phytochemical is found in many peppers, from the mild-tasting bell pepper to the hotter chile pepper to the scorching jalapeño chile pepper. Even the relatively mild and somewhat sweeter paprika pepper contains some capsaicin. The hotter the taste, the more capsaicin the pepper contains. All of these peppers (which technically are berries, not vegetables) belong to the nightshade family. Cayenne, indigenous to the equatorial area of the Americas but now grown in tropical and temperate gardens around the world, is probably the best-known source of the phytochemical capsaicin.

Therapeutic Uses:

ᴥᴥ Arthritis, cramps, menstrual pain, muscle pain, pain.

ᴥ Alcoholism, backache, bursitis, chickenpox, cluster and other headaches, colds, colic, diabetes, diabetic neuropathy, gas, hardening of the arteries, heart disease, high cholesterol, high triglycerides, indigestion, lack of appetite, lumbago, lung problems, nerve pain, pain, shingles, sore throat, sprains, strains, stroke, tennis elbow, thumb sucking, varicose veins.

▦ Folk uses: Chilblains, chills, diarrhea, fever, frostbite, hoarseness, impotence, laryngitis, lumbago, malaria, orgasmic inability, psoriasis, thyroid disease.

Medicinal Properties:

Cayenne and its kin are therapeutic wonders. Their main active ingredient, capsaicin, does far more than force you to gasp for water and make your brow bead with sweat. Applied topically, it works partly as a counterirritant, but it also blocks a body chemical integral to the transmission of pain impulses. Clinical studies have demonstrated its value in alleviating pain and discomfort from rheumatoid arthritis and osteoarthritis, psoriasis, cluster headaches, diabetic neuropathy, mastectomy and breast reconstruction surgery, and shingles. It also significantly cuts the pain from mouth sores associated with chemotherapy and radiation. Salicylates (like those in aspirin) add to its pain-preventing power.

Internally, capsaicin, by reducing both cholesterol and triglycerides, helps keep the blood flowing freely and smoothly through veins and arteries. It also cuts compounds that thicken blood and encourage clotting. Antioxidant nutrients in peppers enhance their cardiovascular protection. The antioxidants guard your lungs, too, and the capsaicin thins mucus, allowing you to expel it more easily. Capsaicin and other phytochemical compounds in pepper plants fight bacteria and muscle spasms. They relieve gas, accentuate the action of digestive enzymes, and open bronchial passages.

And if you're wondering why hot peppers are so popular in hot areas of the Americas, here's a clue: Although they taste hot, the peppers in fact trigger the "cooling center" of your brain's hypothalamus, thus lowering body temperature.

Prescription Counterparts:

Cayenne and capsaicin are solidly established in over-the-counter and prescription-strength pain preparations (such as Zostrix and Dolorac). These products are likely safer than some nonsteroidal anti-inflammatory drugs (NSAIDs) for arthritis pain and myalgia and safer than acyclovir (Zovirax) or famciclovir (Famvir) for shingles.

Dosage Options:

A 450-milligram capsule of a standardized extract three times a day or ¼ to ½ dropper of a tincture daily. You can, of course, also eat as many hot peppers as your mouth can stand or mix ¼ to ½ teaspoon of cayenne pepper in a cup of water and drink it after meals. For a topical ointment, look for a product that contains between 0.025 to 0.075 percent capcaisin. Be extremely careful if you use preparations containing greater amounts.

Safety Rating: 2

Precautions:
For most of us, the worst side effect might be the oral inferno. For a few others, prolonged heavy consumption might cause stomach, liver, or kidney problems. Excessive long-term use also might enhance the effects of blood pressure drugs or other monoamine oxidase inhibitors (MAOIs) or weaken the effectiveness of other drugs. Topically, allergic reactions are rare, but don't rub a capsaicin-containing cream on broken skin or around your eyes or mucous membranes.

CELERY SEED *(Apium graveolens)*

What It Is:
If you've ever crunched your way through a salad or sipped some soup, chances are you've tasted celery's mild flavor. The original plant, wild celery, which grows throughout southern Europe, imparted an acrid, unpleasant taste until seventeenth-century Italian farmers developed what we now call celery and a variant called celeriac, which has an edible root. Celery stalks are good medicine, but the seeds may be even better.

Therapeutic Uses:
〜〜 High blood pressure, water retention.
〜 Anxiety, arthritis, cystitis, gout, heart disease, high cholesterol, insomnia, stress, urinary tract infections.
▦ Folk uses: Depression, diabetes, epilepsy, gallstones, gas, indigestion, lack of appetite, liver problems, kidney stones, menstrual irregularities.

Medicinal Properties:
This unassuming vegetable is another phytochemical powerhouse. The apigenin in celery seeds relaxes blood vessels, allowing them to open wider and permit a freer flow of blood. This is one of more than a dozen chemicals in celery seeds that help your cardiovascular system. Some are natural diuretics, gently encouraging your body to excrete excess fluids, which thwarts high blood pressure and congestive heart failure (as well as monthly premenstrual water retention). Other chemicals act like natural calcium channel blockers and cardiac rhythm stabilizers, making them valuable against an irregular heartbeat or the chest pains of angina. Still other phytochemicals, including a compound called 3-n-butyl-phthalide, help reduce cholesterol and contribute to good blood sugar balance. Celery seed extracts offer some 25 anti-inflammatory substances, which may aid anyone with arthritis. Additional compounds quell spasms and fight a variety of bacteria (notably in the urinary tract). The phthalides in celery seed oil also have a mild sedative effect. And celery seed juice encourages bile production, which improves digestion.

Prescription Counterparts:
Mainstream medicine's answer to gout prevention is allopurinol, a drug well-known to cause skin reactions, diarrhea, drowsiness, and nausea. Conventional doctors like to prescribe diuretics for high blood pressure and water retention, but these have many possible side effects: They can deplete the body of trace minerals and other essential nutrients, raise blood sugar and blood fats, elevate levels of gout-causing uric acid, and disturb the heart's natural rhythm. In Great Britain, celery seeds are an ingredient in more than 50 anti-inflammatory products.

Dosage Options:
Two 500-milligram capsules of a standardized extract once or twice a day before meals, 1 to 2 teaspoons of whole seeds (or ¾ teaspoon crushed) in a cup of hot water daily, or ½ to 1 teaspoon of celery seed tincture up to three times a day. You're also welcome to munch on as many celery stalks as you'd like.

Safety Rating: 2

Precautions:
The overwhelming majority of people will suffer no side effects. A few hypersensitive people might experience an instantaneous allergic reaction. A few others might become more sensitive to sunlight. Researchers have documented one case in which a woman suffered a severe phototoxic reaction after eating some celeriac and then sitting in a tanning booth. Oils in the plant also might exacerbate kidney inflammation, but such cases are uncommon. Lab experiments suggest that the oils could provoke uterine contractions. Lastly, a few people have an allergy called birch-celery syndrome. If you're sensitive to birch or mugwort pollen, you may have an immediate reaction to celery.

CHAMOMILE, GERMAN *(Matricaria recutita;* previously, *Chamomilla recutita)*

What It Is:
Nature grows two different chamomiles—German chamomile and Roman chamomile *(Anthemis nobilis)*. To an amateur, they're almost indistinguishable from each other. Their flowers resemble daisies, with yellow centers and white petals, and both have down-covered stems and fine, feathery, light green leaves. Both also smell a little like apple. For medicinal purposes, you might prefer the German version, an annual that was introduced to North America from Europe and now occasionally grows wild from the northern East Coast and Newfoundland as far west as Minnesota. It's also known as Hungarian chamomile, common chamomile, and wild chamomile.

Therapeutic Uses:

🌿🌿 Bedsores, breathing problems, bruises, bug bites, burns, colds, coughing, fever, frostbite, gallbladder problems, gas, gastritis, gum disease, hemorrhoids, indigestion, insomnia, liver problems, mouth inflammation, skin irritations, sore throat, varicose veins, wounds.

🌿 Acne, allergies, anxiety, arthritis, breast pain, bunions, colic, cramps, diarrhea, earache, eczema, flu, gout, infections, inflammation, lack of menstruation, motion sickness, radiation exposure, rectal inflammation (proctitis), sciatica, sores, stomach problems, sunburn, tissue swelling, toothache, ulcers, vaginal discharge, water retention, yeast infections.

▦ Folk uses: Bloating, cancer, canker sores, colitis, convulsions, dental infections.

Medicinal Properties:

Chamomile extract displays a wide range of therapeutic powers. It's anti-inflammatory, antibacterial, antifungal, antiseptic, antispasmodic, and even anti–body odor. It fights water retention, keeps blood from becoming too viscous, calms edgy nerves, relaxes muscles, boosts the immune system, and reduces intestinal gas. In scientists' never-ending quest for a "silver bullet," they have tried to isolate the single most active substance in chamomile, with apigenin and other flavones, chamazulene, and a-bisabolol often identified. But most studies have concluded that a whole-herb extract is better than any individual phytochemicals.

Prescription Counterparts:

In Europe, chamomile oil is incorporated into a number of over-the-counter anti-inflammatories and antiseptics. On this side of the Atlantic, you'll have to go to a health food store to find chamomile-containing products (check the labels). Research has determined that the plant's apigenin is three times as effective as the opioid analgesic drug papaverine, which can cause liver problems. It's also a better anti-inflammatory than indomethacin. Tested against hydrocortisone, chamomile extract proved superior for easing skin inflammation and just as good for treating eczema. And if you're wondering how well the herb works as a sedative, consider the study in which oral doses of an extract induced deep sleep in 10 out of 12 people who underwent cardiac catheterization.

Dosage Options:

Two or three 350-milligram capsules three times a day, 2 to 3 teaspoons of dried chamomile flowers in a cup of hot water, ½ to 1 teaspoon of chamomile tincture up to three times a day, or ¼ to 1 teaspoon of a liquid extract three times a day. You can apply chamomile poultices directly to inflamed muscles and joints. To prevent and treat gum disease, try gargling with chamomile tea.

Safety Rating: 3

Precautions:
None reported. If you're allergic to ragweed pollen, you might suffer a cross-reaction upon ingestion (or inhalation) of chamomile pollen. Those who are extremely sensitive to chamomile also may experience a cross-reaction with celery or aster-family herbs. Some other phytochemicals in the plant might prompt an allergic reaction in a few people. Excessive consumption of large amounts may induce vomiting or uterine contractions. The natural coumarin in chamomile may enhance the action of blood thinners.

CHAPARRAL *(Larrea tridentata)*

What It Is:
This is one tough shrub, able to survive without water for quite some time in its native southwestern desert areas of the United States. When the rain arrives, it flourishes. Its small yellow flowers bloom, and its leaves weep a sticky resin that smells like creosote or tar. (That's why locals in the desert call it creosote bush.) In Mexico, it's called *hediondilla,* which translates as "little stinker."

Therapeutic Uses:
⌒ Infections, parasitic infections, skin cancer, yeast infections.
▨ Folk uses: Acne, alcoholism, arthritis, bowel cramps, bronchitis, burns, colds, diarrhea, obesity, pain, snakebite, tuberculosis, venereal disease.

Medicinal Properties:
Certain phytochemicals in chaparral oppose free radical oxidation, quell spasms, and kill bacteria. The lignans destroy amoebas and fungi. A few studies have investigated the plant's use against cancer, but results have been mixed.

Dosage Options:
If you're inspired to try chaparral, which is readily available at health food stores, think twice.

Safety Rating:
Do not use.

Precautions:
Chaparral has been linked to liver inflammation; don't use it if you have cirrhosis or another liver disease. It also might cause nausea, fever, and jaundice (including symptoms such as dark urine and a yellowish discoloration of the eyes). Direct contact with the plant might provoke a skin reaction in some sensitive people.

CHASTEBERRY *(Vitex agnus-castus)*

What It Is:
Chasteberry may actually deserve its name. This deciduous shrub native to the Mediterranean region, with its lancelike leaves, fragrant flowers, and gray or purple berries that look a little like peppercorns, has a long reputation for treating menstrual disorders. It's particularly noted for putting the brakes on libido, hence this common name and another: monk's pepper.

Therapeutic Uses:
👄👄 Acne, breast milk deficiency, breast pain, menstrual irregularities (either a dearth or an excess of menstrual flow), premenstrual tension.
👄 Cramps, depression, endometriosis, fibrocystic breast disease, headache, herpes, infertility, menopause, menstrual irregularities, mouth problems, neuroses, prostate enlargement (benign), stomach problems, uterine fibroids, vaginal problems, yeast infections.
▦ Folk uses: Dementia, epilepsy, impotence, orgasmic inability, retarded sexual maturity.

Medicinal Properties:
Research suggests that chasteberry works primarily on the pituitary gland to stabilize and balance the hormonal fluctuations that women experience every month. By increasing the body's secretion of luteinizing hormone, it reduces prolactin and increases both progesterone and follicle-stimulating hormone. Amenorrhea (the absence of menstruation) frequently coincides with higher blood concentrations of prolactin, and prolactin-lowering medications typically normalize the monthly cycle. That's what chasteberry does, as demonstrated in a small study of 20 women with amenorrhea who took 40 drops of chasteberry extract every day. Of the 15 who went the distance in this 6-month experiment, 10 regained their menstrual regularity. A little evidence suggests that chasteberry flowers contain the plant world's equivalent of human testosterone, which would theoretically stimulate, rather than deter, sexual desire. Other compounds in the berries counteract bacteria and fungi, notably candidas.

Dosage Options:
Two 560-milligram capsules twice a day, or try 30 to 40 milligrams of dried berries (or 20 milligrams of the fresh fruit), ¼ to 1 teaspoon of a liquid extract, or ¼ to 1 teaspoon of chasteberry tincture daily.

Safety Rating: 2

Precautions:
None reported for the vast majority of people. Some people might notice a skin reaction or a little gastric upset. Because it influences the body's hormonal balance, chasteberry could interfere with sex-related medications, including oral contracep-

tives and hormone replacement therapy. You might want to think twice about chasteberry if depression is a prominent part of your monthly premenstrual tension. Some scientists have pointed to an increase in progesterone as the culprit in the mood dip.

CHICKWEED *(Stellaria media)*

What It Is:
One of the most common weeds in the world, chickweed grows throughout temperate North America (and even the Arctic), although it originated in Europe. The plant is an annual, with long, tangling stems, oval leaves, and minute white flowers that open in the sun but often close on overcast or rainy days. Birds love the seeds that emerge from the flowers. When boiled, leaves from young plants supposedly taste like spring spinach. Fresh chickweed greens have long been a favorite in salads.

Therapeutic Uses:
Folk uses: Abscesses, arthritis, asthma, boils, breathing problems, bug bites, conjunctivitis, constipation, coughing, dermatitis, diarrhea, eczema, fever, gout, hemorrhoids, inflammation, itching, lung disorders, obesity, psoriasis, sores, sore throat, tuberculosis, ulcers, wounds.

Medicinal Properties:
Chickweed's inflammation-cooling properties have never been validated scientifically, but that hasn't stopped herbal advocates from using it as an anti-inflammatory, whether for internal or external flare-ups. Compounds in the plant also help you to digest food and cough up mucus. The saponins in chickweed improve the absorption of topically applied substances and may even speed the internal absorption of medications.

Dosage Options:
Three 389-milligram capsules or as much as ¼ to ½ cup of the fresh herb three times a day, or try 6 to 12 grams of the dried herb, ¼ to 1 teaspoon of a tincture, or ¼ to 1 teaspoon of a liquid extract daily. Try a chickweed poultice on an abscess, carbuncle, or other external inflammatory sore. And don't forget to try chickweed in a salad.

Safety Rating: 2

Precautions:
None reported, save for a sole case of supposed nitrate toxicity.

CHICORY (Cichorium intybus)

What It Is:
If coffee isn't your cup of tea, perhaps chicory is more to your liking. It's an excellent caffeine-free substitute for java. In fact, several canned brands of coffee contain roasted chicory root (check the labels). Although you're probably familiar with chicory as a coffee additive, you're probably not familiar with it as a plant. Introduced to the United States and southern Canada from Europe, it will grow almost anywhere, although it prefers a humid climate. Herbalists like to dig up the roots, but you should first stop and appreciate its pretty pale blue flowers. You're even less likely to know that chicory is an industrial source of fructose and a sugar enhancer called maltol.

Therapeutic Uses:
ᴥᴥ Gallbladder inflammation, indigestion, lack of appetite, liver problems.
ᴥ Bacterial infections, constipation, heart disease, high blood sugar, high cholesterol, inflammation, irregular heart rhythm, rapid heart rate, swelling, water retention.
▨ Folk uses: Arthritis, cancer, dermatitis, gout, jaundice.

Medicinal Properties:
Consider chicory if you have a liver or heart problem. In one lab test, chicory extract prevented death in mice that were loaded up with lethal doses of acetaminophen. (In high doses, acetaminophen is toxic to the liver.) Some 70 percent of the chicory-eating mice survived the deliberate overdose. All the mice that did not ingest chicory died. Chicory also could be our best source of inulin, a phytochemical that bucks up the immune system, leading it to speed white blood cells to infectious sites. Its cichoric acid also stimulates the immune system. Other compounds in the plant fight inflammation and bacterial infections to a limited extent. In addition, they deter water retention, counter constipation, and help lower cholesterol and blood sugar.

Prescription Counterparts:
Conventional cardiologists often prescribe digitalis to stimulate the heart. You shouldn't medicate yourself if you have a heart problem, but an experienced herbal physician might include chicory as part of a natural complement of herbs to help treat heart disease and wean you off pharmaceuticals.

Dosage Options:
Three to 5 grams of powered chicory root or 3 grams of fresh roots daily.

Safety Rating: 3

Precautions:
A few people could be oversensitive to chicory, as well as to other plants in the Asteraceae family. Other people could develop a skin reaction to the plant. Further digging unearths the case of a vegetable wholesaler who suffered an allergic reaction after ingesting, inhaling, or even touching chicory. (The wholesaler also reacted after eating endive, a botanical relative of chicory, and lettuce.) Most people won't have any problems.

CINNAMON (Cinnamomum verum) AND CASSIA (C. aromaticum)

What It Is:
These two different plants are virtually indistinguishable in looks, flavor, and chemistry. Spice dealers lump cinnamon and cassia together when they dry and powder the plants' bark; medical researchers probably haven't bothered to distinguish between the two either. To split hairs, cassia is also called Chinese cinnamon, false cinnamon, bastard cinnamon, and Canton cassia. It's native to southern China, Vietnam, and Burma. This plant has small flowers arranged in trios and a pea-size fruit. Its flowers, bark, and bark oil contain the medicinal wallop. "Real" cinnamon is indigenous to southwestern India and Sri Lanka. It features tiny, white green flowers with a disagreeable scent and oval fruit that resemble berries. The natural medicine is contained primarily in the bark of younger trees and the oil squeezed from the bark and leaves.

Therapeutic Uses:
🐛🐛 Bronchitis, colds, coughing, fever, gas, indigestion, infections, intestinal spasms, lack of appetite, oral inflammation, sore throat.
🐛 Colic, diarrhea, hemorrhage, intestinal pain, menstrual pain and irregularities, pain, ulcers, yeast infections.
▦ Folk uses: Arthritis, chills, conjunctivitis, flu, nerve pain, orgasmic inability, toothache, uterine relaxation, vaginitis, worms, wounds.

Medicinal Properties:
The phytochemical compounds in cinnamon and cassia ease allergies, reduce pain, counteract bacteria and fungi (including candidas), disinfect wounds, quell spasms and help relax muscles, relieve gas, perk up the movement of food through your intestinal tract, and beat back bugs and other insects.

Dosage Options:
Besides a sprinkle in your applesauce or on top of your toast, try 1 teaspoon of cinnamon in a cup of hot water two or three times a day with meals. Or try ½ to 1 milliliter of a liquid extract, ½ to 1 teaspoon of cinnamon tincture, or 0.3 to 1 gram of powdered bark.

Safety Rating: 3

Precautions:
Only a handful of extremely sensitive people will have a negative reaction to cinnamon, typically contact dermatitis (perhaps a rash, burning, itching, or swollen lips or tongue). If you're this sensitive, avoid perfumes, cosmetics, ointments, mouthwashes, and toothpastes that contain this spice. In one experiment, very high doses of cinnamon caused dogs to vomit. Cinnamon and one of its active ingredients, cinnamaldehyde, might weaken the effect of tetracycline.

CLEAVERS *(Galium aparine)*

What It Is:
Cleavers is a coffee relative, and its seeds, if roasted lightly, are a caffeine-free, albeit inferior, substitute for the traditional morning eye-opener. It grows in moist soil throughout North and South America and the vaguely defined area between Europe and Asia. The bristle-covered fruit emerging from its whitish or green flowers will latch onto (cleave to, if you will) animals that brush by—hence one of the plant's other names, catchweed. Because geese like it a lot, it's also called goosegrass.

Therapeutic Uses:
🍃 Burns, constipation, cystitis, dermatitis, enlarged lymph glands, hemorrhage, high blood pressure, urinary tract infections, venereal disease, yeast infections.
▦ Folk uses: Cancer, fever, jaundice, kidney stones, nerve problems, psoriasis, sores, ulcers, urinary problems, wounds.

Medicinal Properties:
In one study involving dogs, a cleavers extract lowered blood pressure without slowing heart rate or having any health-threatening side effects. The asperuloside in cleavers is a mild laxative.

Dosage Options:
One ounce of dried leaves in a pint of water, 1 to 2 teaspoons of cleavers tincture, 2 to 4 grams of the dried herb in a cup of boiling water, or ½ to 1 teaspoon of a liquid extract three times a day.

Safety Rating: 2

Precautions:
Most people won't encounter any problems. If you have diabetes, ingest cleavers juice cautiously.

CLOVE *(Syzygium aromaticum)*

What It Is:
For both culinary and medicinal purposes, clove has been around since before Christ's birth. At first available only in the East, clove became one of the hottest commodities among early European traders. Today the evergreen is grown in, among other countries, Brazil, Jamaica, Tanzania, and Indonesia. Its shiny leaves are covered with fragrance-releasing glands, but its small flowers, which are what you have in your spice rack, are even more aromatic. (Actually, you don't have the flowers in your flavor arsenal; you have the buds that were picked and dried before blooming.) Clove oil is also extracted from the buds.

Therapeutic Uses:
🌿🌿 Athlete's foot, bronchitis, colds, coughing, fever, infections, inflammation, mouth inflammation, pain, pharyngitis, toothache.
🌿 Bad breath, bug bites, bunions, colic, dermatitis, diarrhea, gum problems, macular degeneration, sores, vaginitis, wounds, yeast infections.
▩ Folk use: Sore throat.

Medicinal Properties:
Clove's healthful help comes courtesy of eugenol, a powerful, multifaceted phytochemical that anesthetizes, kills bacteria and fungi, fights free radical oxidation, and thins the blood. Clove oil is virtually pure eugenol. It deadens pain (particularly in teeth), destroys bacteria (including the little bugs that cause bad breath and infect cuts and scrapes), and helps protect the retina from macular degeneration. Applied topically, it may even alleviate bunion pain.

Prescription Counterparts:
Clove is the active ingredient in many over-the-counter mouthwashes and preparations designed to ease tooth pain (check the labels). Your dentist may use clove oil as both an anesthetic and an antiseptic.

Dosage Options:
One hundred to 300 milligrams of powdered cloves daily. For bad breath, make a tea with 1 to 2 teaspoons of the dried herb and drink daily. Make your own mouthwash by steeping several tablespoons of powdered cloves in a pint of vodka for a few days. For a cut, sprinkle on a little powdered cloves to prevent infection. For a toothache, rub a little clove oil directly where it hurts, but don't drink the straight oil.

Safety Rating: 3

Precautions:
None reported, although the eugenol in clove oil can irritate the skin or mouth. Some suggest that clove could interfere with blood thinners. An advisory panel to the FDA, however, endorsed clove oil as the safest and most effective active ingredient in toothache remedies.

COFFEE *(Coffea arabica)*

What It Is:
Coffee is probably the most popular drug in the world. This densely leaved shrub with its aromatic white flowers and reddish brown berries originally came from what is now Ethiopia, and by the fifteenth century or so, it was cultivated in various parts of the Middle East. The reputation of the invigorating brew spread from there, and a couple of hundred years later, drinking coffee was in vogue in Europe. For a long time, Arab lands controlled the plant and its seeds, with most of the world's coffee supply being shipped through the port of Mocha. In the late 1600s, Dutch traders smuggled some seeds out of the area and cultivated them on the Indonesian island of Java, giving rise to another name for the brew. From there, the plant was introduced to Central America, Brazil, Jamaica, and elsewhere.

Therapeutic Uses:
🌿🌿 Diarrhea, dizziness, oral inflammation, sore throat.
🌿 Asthma, bronchitis, flu, hepatitis, lung disease, migraine, sleepiness, stomach acid insufficiency, water retention, wounds.

Medicinal Properties:
Coffee is so ingrained in cultures around the world that you'd be hard-pressed to find someone who doesn't know that coffee owes its main therapeutic effect—stimulation of the central nervous system—to the phytochemical caffeine, the prime ingredient in tea, certain colas, cocoa, and chocolate. Caffeine perks you up in several ways: It accelerates the heart, increases blood flow, and encourages breathing. But this phytochemical doesn't deserve all the accolades. Other substances in coffee, including theobromine and theophylline, help expand lung passages and inhibit bronchospasms. Another phytochemical, chlorogenic acid, can get your gastric juices flowing. See page 17 for why coffee is this book's benchmark for herbal safety.

Dosage Options:
Just make a cup—or a whole pot. Everyone has his or her own preference for how strong a cup of joe should be. Add a little honey and some milk for taste. Three average cups will provide anywhere from 250 to 500 milligrams of caffeine.

Safety Rating: 2

Precautions:
Don't drink a cup of coffee before you go to bed; it could prevent you from falling asleep. Chronic, excessive consumption at any time of day also could prevent you from falling asleep at night, make you irritable and restless, prompt heart palpitations, raise cholesterol and blood pressure, upset your stomach, or aggravate kidney

problems. Nursing moms who drink coffee might transfer the caffeine to their babies, agitating them and giving them insomnia. Don't down your mineral supplements with your morning brew. Coffee may impede your body's absorption of calcium, magnesium, iron, and other nutrients. It also might interfere with the absorption of certain medications.

COLA (*Cola*, various species)

What It Is:
When the soft drink industry was in its infancy, Coca-Cola contained a large amount of this tree's nuts (not to mention coca leaf and cocaine). Today soft drinks contain little, if any, true cola. But people in West Africa, where the tree is native, still enjoy the real thing, as do those in Indonesia, Brazil, and the other tropical lands in which more than 100 different species grow. The cola tree features long, leathery leaves and small yellow flowers from which brown pods grow. The cola nuts (which actually are seeds) are nestled inside the pods.

Therapeutic Uses:
🍃🍃 Fatigue.
🍃 Asthma, diarrhea, dysentery, exhaustion, headache, lack of appetite, lethargy, migraine, nerve pain.
▦ Folk uses: Depression, indigestion, inflammation, melancholy, morning sickness, wounds.

Medicinal Properties:
Like coffee, cola contains caffeine and theobromine, both central nervous system stimulants. (See "Coffee" on page 78.)

Dosage Options:
One to 2 teaspoons of powdered cola nuts in a cup of hot water up to three times a day, up to 1 dropper of cola nut tincture or concentrate daily, or ½ to a little more than 1 teaspoon of a liquid extract daily.

Safety Rating: 2

Precautions:
Cola is generally safe. (See the precautions under "Coffee" on page 78.)

COLEUS FORSKOHLII *(Plectranthus barbatus)*

What It Is:
Grown along mountain slopes in India, Nepal, Thailand, and Sri Lanka, coleus forskohlii, also called coleus, has been used for centuries in Ayurvedic medicine. Only this species of the mint-family perennial contains, in its roots, the active compound forskolin.

Therapeutic Uses:
✿ Asthma, congestive heart failure, glaucoma, heart disease, high blood pressure, ischemia.

▦ Folk uses: Convulsions, eczema, hypothyroidism, indigestion, infertility, insomnia, psoriasis, respiratory problems, skin problems.

Medicinal Properties:
Even though coleus has a long history in folk medicine, its phytochemical secret, forskolin, was discovered only in 1974. Several thousand laboratory studies have since been conducted on this chemical. The compound has a vast range of effects on the body, working primarily on an enzymatic level. It triggers adenylate cyclase, which then raises the level of cyclic AMP (adenosine 3',5'-monophosphate), a substance that activates all sorts of other cellular enzymes. Researchers suspect that lowered cyclic AMP production contributes significantly to a number of health problems, including asthma, the chest pains of angina, eczema, high blood pressure, psoriasis, and a number of inflammatory conditions. Higher cell concentrations of this substance reduce inflammation and histamine release, improve the heart's ability to contract, relax arteries and other smooth muscles (including in the lungs, intestinal tract, and bladder), and boost the body's production of both insulin and thyroid hormone. Studies have demonstrated that pharmaceutical forskolin preparations accomplish all these things. It also improves blood flow inside the brain and eases the intraocular pressure of glaucoma by stimulating better blood flow inside the eyes. Other research suggests that potential benefits of forskolin include help in losing weight, improving digestion and nutrient absorption, fighting cancer, and bolstering the immune system.

Dosage Options:
The whole root contains only a minute amount of forskolin and thus may not provide a therapeutic response. The isolated chemical is a prescription medication. One possible option is to ingest 6 to 12 grams of dried coleus root a day; better to stick with a supplement standardized for its forskolin content. Look for a product containing 18 percent forskolin; a typical dose is 50 milligrams (which will provide about 9 milligrams of the active phytochemical) two or three times a day. The standardized supplement, unlike the isolated drug, should contain various helper phytochemicals that improve forskolin's performance and absorption.

Safety Rating: 2

Precautions:
Be wary if you have hypotension, because coleus may reduce blood pressure even more. Supplements also may strengthen the action of certain prescription drugs, notably those used to treat asthma and high blood pressure.

COLTSFOOT *(Tussilago farfara)*

What It Is:
If you're up on your Latin, you know that this perennial's generic first name means "cough." In fact, it once was called coughwort. Coltsfoot earned its current moniker because its broad, serrated leaves are shaped somewhat like a colt's foot. Interestingly, the leaves don't emerge until after the appearance of its yellow flowers, which look like dandelions. Originating in Europe, the plant now pops up in damp areas from Newfoundland south to New Jersey and Maryland and west to Minnesota.

Therapeutic Uses:
🌿🌿 Bronchitis, colds, coughing, hoarseness, mouth inflammation, mucous membrane inflammation, pharyngitis, respiratory problems.
🌿 Asthma, laryngitis.
▦ Folk uses: Congestion, diarrhea, flu, lung problems, lymph gland enlargement or disease, sore throat, tonsillitis, whooping cough.

Medicinal Properties:
Since the days of ancient Greece and Rome, coltsfoot has been eaten, drunk, and even smoked to relieve asthma, hacking, and bronchial congestion. Its active ingredients help break up mucus and expel it from your respiratory system. It also hinders the body's production of an inflammatory protein called platelet-activating factor, which narrows the air passages and prompts asthma attacks.

Dosage Options:
Two teaspoons of powdered leaves steeped in a cup of hot water daily, ⅛ to ½ teaspoon of a liquid leaf extract three times a day, ½ to a little more than 1 teaspoon of coltsfoot tincture three times a day, or ⅛ to ½ teaspoon of a liquid flower extract once a day.

Safety Rating: 1

Precautions:
Used judiciously for short periods, coltsfoot should cause no problems; consult a qualified physician. But that view is not universally shared among herbal experts. The plant contains substances called pyrrolizidine alkaloids (PAs), which are toxic to the liver. The American Herbal Products Association recommends that all products containing PAs carry a statement warning that they are for external use only,

should not be applied to broken or abraded skin, and should not be used when pregnant or while nursing. Ingesting 0.5 to 3.3 milligrams for every 2.2 pounds of body weight was found to be severely or fatally toxic. A standard cup of coltsfoot tea, containing 2 to 3 teaspoons of powdered leaves, provides a level of PAs (about 10 milligrams) that Germany's Commission E has deemed safe for occasional use.

COMFREY (*Symphytum*, various species)

What It Is:
The name comfrey apparently was derived from a Latin word that translates as "knitting together." Over the ages, it's also been known as bruisewort, knitback, and knitbone. All these aliases contain a clue to its therapeutic use. Another onetime name, ass ear, is more of a tip-off to what the plant's long green leaves look like. Originally found only in Eurasia, comfrey, with its bell-shaped purple flowers, now grows wild in the eastern United States and Canada.

Therapeutic Uses:
 Bruises, joint sprains, ulcers (duodenal and indolent).
 Arthritis, bedsores, breast pain, bronchitis, bug bites, chafing, colitis, eczema, fractures, gastritis, gum disease, hemorrhage, inflammation, intestinal inflammation, muscle strains, pharyngitis, psoriasis, rashes, sores, wounds.
 Folk uses: Chest pain, congestion, contusions, coughing, diarrhea, dysentery, gastric ulcers, indigestion, itching, pleuritis, sunburn, venous problems.

Medicinal Properties:
One of the main therapeutic substances in comfrey is allantoin, an anti-inflammatory that perks up the immune system, speeds wound healing, and encourages new skin and cell growth. It's a time-honored treatment for healing sores, bruises, and even broken bones. The tannins in comfrey are astringent, and the rosmarinic acid might contribute some anti-inflammatory assistance. Some extracts have shown the potential to decrease tumor growth and extend the lives of lab mice with cancer.

Prescription Counterparts:
A doctor probably would prescribe antibiotics for diabetes-related sores. In consultation with your physician, you might want to try comfrey instead. You'll find comfrey or allantoin in several readily available skin creams (check the labels).

Dosage Options:
Two to 4 grams of dried roots or 2 to 8 grams of dried leaves in a tea three times a day, ½ to 1 teaspoon of a liquid extract three times a day, or ¼ to ½ cup of fresh comfrey leaves daily. To apply topically as a poultice or compress, mix powdered comfrey with a little vegetable oil and make a paste. Or mash the plant's fresh leaves.

Safety Rating: 1

Precautions:
Not for long-term internal consumption—in reasonable dosages, no longer than a total of 4 to 6 weeks in a year; consult a qualified physician. Like coltsfoot (see the precautions under "Coltsfoot" on page 81), comfrey contains pyrrolizidine alkaloids (PAs), which in excessive amounts have been linked to severe, even lethal, liver toxicity. The warnings have given comfrey a bad rap, and even herbalists are divided on whether to use this age-old herb. Some say that it should be applied only externally; others point to research asserting that a cup of comfrey tea possesses less cancer-causing potential than a can of beer.

CORN SILK *(Zea mays)*

What It Is:
When you husk an ear of corn, you're throwing away a little medicine. Those long, silky threads have traditionally been used in a variety of folk remedies.

Therapeutic Uses:
🌿 Cystitis, gonorrhea, gout, hardening of the arteries, premenstrual tension, prostatitis, tissue swelling, urinary tract inflammation and infections, water retention.
▦ Folk uses: Arthritis, bed-wetting, bladder stones, kidney inflammation, liver problems, urinary problems.

Medicinal Properties:
Extracts of corn silk are potent diuretics, giving rise to their use for all sorts of kidney-related and urinary complaints. The diuretic effect comes in handy for water retention and tissue swelling (whether from PMS or kidney disease), cystitis, urinary infections, or any other inflammation of the urinary tract.

Dosage Options:
Four to 8 grams of dried corn silk brewed into a tea three times a day, ½ to a little more than 1 teaspoon of a liquid extract daily, or 1 teaspoon to 1 tablespoon of corn silk tincture daily.

Safety Rating: 3

Precautions:
Except for a few cases of dermatitis and other allergic reactions, none reported. In rabbits, corn silk has triggered uterine contractions, so you might want to think twice about using it if you're pregnant.

CRANBERRY *(Vaccinium macrocarpum)*

What It Is:
Cranberry bushes feature leathery leaves and bright red berries. The plant grows mostly in peat bogs in eastern North America, from Newfoundland south to North and South Carolina and west to the Midwest. The berries you buy at the supermarket a day or two before Thanksgiving probably were harvested in Massachusetts or Wisconsin.

Therapeutic Uses:
❧❧ Bladder infections, cystitis, kidney inflammation and infections, urinary tract infections, water retention.
▦ Folk use: Gout.

Medicinal Properties:
Cranberry is top-notch "food farmacy"; all you need to do is drink the fruit juice. It is a great antiseptic that prevents bacteria, including E. coli, from clinging to the interior of the bladder. No clinging means no infection. The arbutin in cranberry not only fights infections but also encourages urinary excretion to ease water retention and tissue swelling.

Prescription Counterparts:
Conventional doctors prescribe synthetic bactericides or other antibiotics for urinary infections. Don't rule out pharmaceutical intervention for a urinary tract infection, but you might want to drink a few glasses of 100 percent cranberry juice (see "Precautions") before you go to the doctor and ask for a drug.

Dosage Options:
Two or three 505-milligram capsules of cranberry juice concentrate daily with a meal or 1 tablespoon of the dried fruit in a cup of hot water. To prevent urinary problems, drink at least 3 ounces of 100 percent cranberry juice (see "Precautions") every day. To treat urinary problems, drink 12 to 32 ounces of cranberry juice.

Safety Rating: 3

Precautions:
None reported. If you drink a ridiculous amount—say 3 to 4 quarts of cranberry juice a day—you might get diarrhea or notice some other gastrointestinal upset. Perhaps the biggest precaution is a manufacturing-related one: Look for 100 percent cranberry juice. Avoid the "cocktails" that are diluted and adulterated with sugar or corn syrup.

D

DAMIANA *(Turnera diffusa)*

What It Is:
Folklore and herbal hucksters tout this shrub as an aphrodisiac, particularly for women. Many plant specialists doubt the claim, which has never been proved scientifically. Nonetheless, its reputation is solidly established from centuries of use in Mexico and the southwestern United States, where damiana, with its wedge-shaped leaves and starlike yellow flowers, grows wild.

Therapeutic Uses:
▨ Folk uses: Anxiety, asthma, bed-wetting, colds, constipation, coughing, depression, diabetes, headache, indigestion, kidney inflammation, low libido, menstrual irregularities.

Medicinal Properties:
As noted, damiana's power to perk up a lazy libido has never been validated, but there is encouraging anecdotal evidence. Extracts do display some antibacterial action and have helped lower blood sugar in lab mice.

Dosage Options:
One or two 400-milligram capsules up to three times a day, 1 dropper of damiana tincture daily, or a tea made from 2 to 4 grams of dried damiana shoots three times a day.

Safety Rating: 2

Precautions:
When taken in reasonable amounts, none reported. Extremely high doses might threaten cyanide poisoning, because the plant contains chemicals called cyanogenetic glycosides. The volatile oils extracted from damiana irritate mucous membranes and work as both a diuretic and a laxative.

DANDELION *(Taraxacum officinale)*

What It Is:

In French, dandelion is *pissenlit,* which translates as "piss in bed," a rather vulgar reference to the urinary encouragement of this perennial herb. Blame (or thank) our early European settlers for bringing the dandelion to North America. Native Americans welcomed it readily for all sorts of uses. The roots can be dried, ground up, and brewed like coffee; the jagged leaves can be eaten in salads; and the yellow flowers make a nice wine. Curse their appearance in your finely manicured lawn, but don't deny yourself their phytochemical value.

Therapeutic Uses:

🌢🌢 Bladder stones, bronchitis, gallbladder problems, gas, indigestion, kidney stones, lack of appetite, liver dysfunction, pneumonia, respiratory problems, urinary tract infections.

🌢 Colds, gas, lack of urination (compared to fluid intake), osteoporosis.

▦ Folk uses: Alcoholism, arthritis, breast pain, cirrhosis, constipation, diabetes, eczema, heart disease, gallstones, gastritis, gout, heartburn, hemorrhoids, infections, jaundice, premenstrual tension, skin problems, tonsillitis.

Medicinal Properties:

Though considered an eyesore and a nuisance by many, dandelion actually is a very good source of nourishment and natural medicine. The leaves provide vitamins A and C; the flowers are one of the plant world's better sources of lecithin, a nutrient that elevates the brain's acetylcholine and may play a role in stemming Alzheimer's disease. Lecithin also is good for liver problems, and the plant is a time-honored treatment for jaundice and other hepatic complaints. Dandelion won't cure a urinary tract infection on its own, but it certainly will help you urinate. The more you go to the bathroom, the more likely you are to flush out those bladder-bothering bacteria. Two sets of phytochemicals, eudesmanolides and germacranolides, apparently are responsible. The potassium in dandelion might help, too. And don't neglect dandelion if you're worried about osteoporosis. It's a great source of three bone-building nutrients: boron, calcium, and silicon.

Dosage Options:

Three 515-milligram capsules three times a day, 1 to 3 teaspoons of powdered dandelion root or ½ ounce of dried dandelion leaves steeped in a cup of hot water daily, 1 to 2 teaspoons of dandelion tincture up to three times a day, ¼ to ½ cup of fresh roots daily, or 1 tablespoon of dandelion juice in the morning and evening. For breast pain (and tonsillitis, according to Chinese physicians), apply a syrupy compress made by soaking an ounce or so of minced dandelion roots in 2 to 3 cups of water and boiling off about half the water. Some people think dandelion greens in a salad are delicious; others consider them bitter.

Safety Rating: 3

Precautions:
Virtually none, although some herbalists advise that people with gallstones or biliary obstruction should take dandelion only under a doctor's guidance, because the herb stimulates bile production. A few hypersensitive people might notice some gastric upset or dermatitis. Don't eat dandelions that have been treated with herbicides.

DEVIL'S CLAW *(Harpagophytum procumbens)*

What It Is:
European herbalists became familiar with devil's claw in the 1950s, but this shrublike perennial vine has a long history of use in southern Africa, where it is indigenous. The bitter-tasting roots have been eaten, drunk as both a tea and a tonic, and made into a topical ointment. The plant's large, claw-shaped fruit gives rise to its name.

Therapeutic Uses:
🌿🌿 Arthritis, backache, gallbladder problems, indigestion, lack of appetite, liver problems.
🌿 Allergies, boils, childbirth, headache, heart disease, inflammation, irregular heart rhythm, migraine.
▦ Folk uses: Cancer, fever, fibrositis, gout, heartburn, lumbago, muscle pain, skin problems, sores, ulcers.

Medicinal Properties:
Harpagoside and other phytochemicals in devil's claw have been studied extensively, notably for their analgesic, anti-inflammatory, and cardiovascular effects. The research confirms that plant extracts quell inflammation, stabilize heart rhythm, and stimulate appetite, among other effects, but practical applications in clinical trials have produced mixed results. Some studies have shown a definite improvement in easing arthritis and acute back pain; others have shown little relief.

Dosage Options:
One to 2 teaspoons of fresh roots, 1½ to 3 teaspoons of a liquid extract, 1 to 2 tablespoons of devil's claw tincture, or 1 teaspoon of chopped dried roots in 2 cups of hot water daily.

Safety Rating: 1

Precautions:
Don't take the herb if you have a duodenal or gastric ulcer, because the plant triggers the flow of gastric juices. High doses could interfere with blood pressure, heart, and diabetes medications.

DONG QUAI *(Angelica sinensis)*

What It Is:

In traditional Chinese medicine, only ginseng is more highly prized and esteemed. Perhaps that's because most traditional Chinese physicians are male, and dong quai, also called Chinese angelica, is commonly used for health complaints unique to women. A female Chinese physician might switch the rankings of the two.

At least nine species of angelica, part of the parsley family, exist. They possess different medicinal traits, but the *sinensis* variant is the most valued. Japanese angelica *(A. acutiloba)* is very similar to dong quai. European angelica *(A. archangelica)* is used primarily for infections. American angelica *(A. atropurpurea)* is used mostly for heartburn, flatulence, and colic, but it can be confused with some of the more poisonous species. Most of the research has been conducted on the Chinese and Japanese species. The name dong quai means "proper order," and for thousands of years the dried roots have been used to restore a healthy order to the body.

Therapeutic Uses:

🍂🍂 Aortic inflammation, Buerger's disease (an inflammatory blood vessel disease that can lead to gangrene), cirrhosis and other liver diseases, infertility, menstrual irregularities.

🍂 Allergies, alveolitis (lung inflammation from extreme sensitivity to organic matter), anemia, arthritis, bruises, constipation, hardening of the arteries, heart disease, intestinal pain, irregular heart rhythm, hot flashes, kidney disease, lack of menstruation, liver toxicity, low libido in women, menopause, menstrual pain, muscular cramps, nerve pain, premenstrual tension.

▦ Folk uses: Chest pain, childbirth, eye inflammation, fibrocystic breast disease, high blood pressure, palpitations, pregnancy, stomachache, stroke, tinnitus, tissue swelling, ulcers.

Medicinal Properties:

Dong quai roots are little phytochemical pharmacies. The phytoestrogens work whether the body's natural estrogen concentration needs to be supplemented or constrained, making it a good treatment for a whole spectrum of female health problems, including menstrual disorders, PMS, menopausal symptoms, and uterine cramps. It also relaxes the smooth muscles in and improves blood flow to the uterus (and elsewhere), two reasons this gnarly root helps your cardiovascular health. It dilates smooth muscles in your arteries, allowing them to permit a freer flow of blood throughout the body, and hinders any tendency for the blood to thicken and clot. It also helps regulate the heart's rhythm.

Dong quai's phytochemicals crank up the production of white blood cells in the immune system, strengthen their ability to fend off invaders, and impede the manufacture of allergy-provoking antigens to things such as animal dander, dust, and pollen. Immune enhancement could come into play in cancer prevention or treatment. Other research suggests that the roots assist the liver in ridding the body of toxins and may improve the metabolism of protein if you have kidney disease. They also have the ability to relieve pain, according to some animal research.

Prescription Counterparts:
Synthetic estrogens are used for a host of women's health disorders. Current studies are equivocal, but if the estrogenic action is proved, dong quai might be a safer adjunct that allows you to lessen your reliance on costly pharmaceuticals. It also could supplement, or permit you to reduce the dosages of, drugs to control high blood pressure, irregular heart rhythm, and the chest pains of angina. Some of its phytochemicals may work much like prescription calcium channel blockers.

Dosage Options:
Three 530-milligram capsules three times a day. Or try 1 to 3 tablespoons of fresh dong quai roots, 2 to 6 grams of dried root, or 1 teaspoon to 1 tablespoon of a liquid extract daily.

Safety Rating: 1

Precautions:
Don't take dong quai if you have diarrhea or an acute viral infection, are pregnant, or are prone to heavy menstrual periods.

DRUG ALOE *(Aloe vera)*

See "Aloes" on page 29.

E

ECHINACEA *(Echinacea,* various species*)*

What It Is:
The most frequently used plant among early Native Americans and the most popular herbal supplement in the United States today, echinacea is second only to garlic as the best that nature has to offer. It's the herbal equivalent of vitamin C. Widely used in America during the nineteenth century, the plant was supplanted by synthetic medications in the twentieth century. Laboratory explorers in Europe later picked up the herbal ball that the New World dropped. Thanks to them, we now know that our Native American predecessors were right all along.

Nine species of the plant, also called purple coneflower, grow perennially throughout midwestern North America, as far north as Saskatchewan and as far south as Texas. Three of them—*E. purpurea, E. pallida,* and *E. angustifolia*—are the most used and most studied. The echinacea species can be difficult to tell apart. All have bright, strikingly pretty purple flowers, except for *E. paradoxa,* whose flowers are yellow. *E. angustifolia* has narrow leaves; *E. purpurea* sports wider, serrated leaves. Herbalists argue over which species is best, just as they debate which part of the plant has the most medicinal value. All variants possess phytochemicals that improve the immune system.

Therapeutic Uses:
🌿🌿 Breast pain, bronchitis, burns, colds, coughing, fever, flu, HIV, immune system depression, infections (including listeria, Lyme disease, trichomoniasis, and typhus), meningitis, mouth inflammation, mumps, pharyngitis, respiratory problems, urinary tract infections, white blood cell insufficiency (leukopenia), wounds.
🌿 Abscesses, acne, allergies, arthritis, blood poisoning, boils, cancer, canker sores, carbuncles, chemotherapy, colon cancer, dry eyes, cramps, Crohn's disease, cystitis, dandruff, dental inflammation, dysentery, earache, eczema, gallbladder problems, goiter, gonorrhea, gum disease, headache, herpes, liver cancer, lymph gland enlargement or disease, meningitis, parasitic infections (particularly leishmaniasis), psoriasis, scarlet fever, sinus problems, skin inflammation, sore throat, tonsillitis, toothache, tuberculosis, varicose veins, whooping cough, yeast infections.
▦ Folk uses: Bug bites, diabetes, diphtheria, hemorrhoids, indigestion and other gastric problems, kidney bleeding, measles, migraine, snakebite, spider bites, syphilis.

Medicinal Properties:
As dozens of scientific studies have established, echinacea is a very potent immune system stimulant, a decent fighter of inflammation and viruses, and a mild antiseptic. It muscles up the body's natural defenses in a variety of ways. One phytochemical, inulin, improves the white blood cells' ability to speed to and tackle infections (whether viral, fungal, or bacterial), in part by increasing the level of a substance called properdin. The plant also increases the number of white blood cells in your immune system arsenal and activates them. Caffeic acid, cichoric acid, and echinacin kill viruses much like the body's own bug killer, interferon. The herb also signals the body to release interferon. The overall impact is a great counterattack to everything from colds and flu to yeast and respiratory infections, perhaps even to cancer and HIV.

Prescription Counterparts:
Echinacea is a worthy competitor of all sorts of prescription and over-the-counter nostrums. For bronchitis, you might want to try it before you take atropine (Donnatal), codeine, or dextromethorphan (Sudafed). For a cold or the flu, give it a chance before you resort to acetaminophen or a decongestant. For rhinitis, take some standardized capsules or drink echinacea tinctures and teas before turning to drugs such as cromolyn (Gastrocom) or phenylpropanolamine (Dimetane).

Dosage Options:
A twice-daily dosage of two 500-milligram capsules of echinacea standardized to contain 125 milligrams each of *E. angustifolia* root extract, including at least 3.2 to 4.8 percent echinacoside. That's a real mouthful, but that's how the strongest potencies are measured. Anything less may not work as well. More traditional forms of the plant also will impart some phytochemical medication, such as a tea made from 2 teaspoons of dried roots in a cup of water three times a day, ¼ to ½ teaspoon of echinacea tincture daily, 300 to 400 milligrams of a solid extract up to three times a day, or up to 1 teaspoon of a liquid root extract three times a day. You can also add a dropper of echinacea tincture to teas and other preparations, including poultices, compresses, mouthwashes, and other tinctures.

Some herbalists say that you shouldn't take echinacea for longer than 2 to 8 weeks because your body might get used to it and no longer respond. The jury is still out on this. If you're concerned, try taking it for a week or two, abstaining for a few days, and then repeating the pattern.

Safety Rating: 3

Precautions:
Your tongue might tingle or get numb when you take echinacea, but that's about the worst most of us can expect. Megadoses might slow down, rather than rev up, the immune system. Some herbalists have speculated that the herb might stimulate HIV rather than help the infection. Some people might experience dose-dependent allergic reactions, nausea, vomiting, chills, or fever. Anyone with multiple sclerosis, systemic lupus erythematosus, or another autoimmune disease probably

should avoid taking the herb. Certain species of echinacea could contain very small amounts of pyrrolizidine alkaloids (PAs), which, in excessive concentrations, have been linked to severe (or even lethal) liver toxicity. The levels in this herb are too low to be of any concern.

ELDER, EUROPEAN; ELDERBERRY *(Sambucus nigra)*

What It Is:
Musical instruments, weaving needles, and, of course, elderberry wine all have come from this plant, a member of the honeysuckle family. People have been cultivating this small tree, with its clusters of tiny white flowers and blackish purple berries, probably since prehistoric times. Nine or so different species of elder grow in various parts of North America and Europe. The bark, berries, and flowers all have been used to make tonics said to do everything from induce sweating and treat colds to encourage excretion. Herbal distributors often confuse the different species and call them by different names, but the best (or at least best studied) of the bunch is *S. nigra,* known variously as elder, European elder, elderberry, and black elderberry. Native Americans used *S. canadensis* for the same medicinal purposes, but this species may have a different medicinal impact.

Therapeutic Uses:
🙣🙣 Bronchitis, colds, coughing.
🙣 Breathing problems, flu, herpes, mucous membrane inflammation, sinusitis, sore throat.
▣ Folk uses: Arthritis, boils, bruises, constipation, eczema, fever, headache, laryngitis, obesity, pain, sores, swelling.

Medicinal Properties:
The phytochemicals in European elder are good viral vanquishers, particularly in the respiratory system. In one clinical trial, a standardized herb extract alleviated symptoms and cured 90 percent of the people hit by a 1993 flu outbreak in Israel in just 3 days. Most of their elderberry-free counterparts in the study didn't get better for almost a week. The extract, some research suggests, binds to flu viruses, preventing them from invading cells and replicating. Bioflavonoids in the extract may contribute to the deterrent effect.

Prescription Counterparts:
The compound used in the Israeli study was a refined extract of elderberry. The evidence is still sketchy, but it may work in a fashion similar to the prescription drug zanamivir (Relenza) and other neuraminidase inhibitors.

Dosage Options:
Put 2 teaspoons of dried European elder flowers in a cup of hot water, steep, strain, and drink several times a day. You can also take ½ to 1 teaspoon of a liquid flower extract three times a day or ½ to 2 teaspoons of a liquid whole-herb extract daily.

Safety Rating: 3

Precautions:
None reported with dried fruit and flowers. Raw or unripe parts of the plant contain a chemical called sambunigrin, which can induce diarrhea or vomiting if consumed in excess.

ELECAMPANE *(Inula helenium)*

What It Is:
In the old days, the plant was included in the U.S. Pharmacopeia; too bad it's no longer listed. As a remedy for bronchial congestion, elecampane has been used since ancient Greece and Rome. In the 1800s, the roots of this pretty, perennial garden flower (the blossoms look like dwarf sunflowers, hence one of its common names, wild sunflower) were mixed with sugar, then boiled and made into cough drops. The plant also was deemed a decent digestive aid. Despite all human applications, elecampane probably was brought from Europe to North America for a veterinary purpose: It helps heal skin infections in horses and sheep.

Therapeutic Uses:
🍂 Bronchitis, colds, congestion, coughing, diarrhea, dysentery, gas, indigestion, infections, respiratory problems, worms, yeast infections.
▦ Folk uses: Arthritis, asthma, dermatitis, diabetes, emphysema, gastric disease, heart disease, kidney disease, liver disease, menstrual irregularities, mucous membrane inflammation, nausea, parasitic infections, tuberculosis, urinary tract infections, whooping cough.

Medicinal Properties:
Elecampane, notably the phytochemical inulin, is a pretty good expectorant, assisting users in coughing up phlegm and bronchial congestion. Inulin also aids in maintaining a good balance of intestinal bacteria, helps ensure regular bowel movements, and soothes inflamed tissue. In research involving people (as opposed to laboratory animals), two other phytochemicals, alantolactone and isoalantolactone, proved useful in treating parasitic infections, including roundworm, hookworm, whipworm, and threadworm. Alantolactone and the plant's essential oil also show some anti-inflammatory, immune-stimulating, and antiseptic (especially against bacteria, fungi, and candidas) qualities.

Dosage Options:
Three hundred milligrams of pure alantolactone every day for 5 days, followed by a 10-day respite and then another 5-day course. Other options include ¼ teaspoon of powdered root in a cup of hot water up to three times a day, ¼ to 1 teaspoon of a liquid root extract, or 1 to 2 teaspoons of fresh roots. If you make elecampane into a tea, make sure you have some honey, licorice, lemon, or sugar on hand; the herb is bitter.

Safety Rating: 2

Precautions:
In large doses, elecampane can cause diarrhea, vomiting, cramps, spasms, or even symptoms of paralysis. In a few very sensitive people, it might prompt an allergic skin reaction. When given to lab mice, the herb worked as a sedative. In other animal experiments, small dosages lowered blood sugar; larger amounts raised blood sugar and lowered blood pressure.

EPHEDRA; MA HUANG (*Ephedra*, various species)

What It Is:
Whether you call it by its American or Chinese name, this controversial plant is one of the oldest known medicines. Herbalists in China have used it for thousands of years. Ephedra is a primitive, almost leafless shrub with minute, yellow green flowers. A number of species grow all over the world, mostly in deserts. The North American variants do not contain the medicinal compounds found in those native to China.

Therapeutic Uses:
🌿🌿 Allergies, asthma, bronchial spasms, bronchitis, colds, coryza (inflammation of the nose with excessive nasal discharge), coughing, respiratory problems, sinusitis.
🌿 Bed-wetting, chest congestion, flu, incontinence, lethargy, low blood pressure, myasthenia gravis, nasal congestion, obesity.
▨ Folk uses: Fever, hay fever, headache, hives.

Medicinal Properties:
Ephedra works, but too well and with too many side effects to regard it as safe for self-medication (see "Precautions"). Its active ingredients, ephedrine and pseudoephedrine, are strong bronchial dilators and decongestants. They narrow blood vessels and constrict other smooth muscles, which is why they're used to treat bed-wetting and low blood pressure. They also stimulate the central nervous system (almost like an amphetamine) and make you sweat, two reasons this herb is so widely promoted as a stimulant and a weight loss aid.

Prescription Counterparts:
Ephedra is, essentially, prescription medication. Pseudoephedrine is the active ingredient in Sudafed and other decongestants. Ephedrine hydrochloride is commonly found not only in health food stores but at truck stops in various parts of the country.

Dosage Options:
Not for self-medication.

Safety Rating:
Do not use except under the advice of a knowledgeable health practitioner.

Precautions:
A handful of people have died over the past few years from abusing ephedra products, prompting the FDA to issue warnings against their use and to consider banning the substance entirely. Even though Germany's Commission E has approved ephedra for respiratory problems, the concern is well-founded. The herb and its extracts are potentially addictive, and they can disrupt regular heart rhythm, induce cardiac arrest, and raise blood pressure. They're likely to make you irritable, nervous, and nauseous. They're also very likely to make you sweat profusely, decrease your appetite, and prevent you from falling asleep. Anyone with high blood pressure, anorexia or bulimia, or diabetes-induced glaucoma should be particularly cautious. Actually, everyone should be cautious: Do not take this herb or its derivatives.

EUCALYPTUS *(Eucalyptus globulus)*

What It Is:
Eucalyptus, a genus with some 500 species, is one of the tallest trees in the world. Some species—indigenous to Australia but now found in various parts of North America, South America, Europe, Africa, and India—can grow up to 300 feet tall. The trees suck up so much water that they are said to eradicate malaria-infested swamps, although that attribute is more often ascribed to the melaleuca (see "Tea Tree" on page 212), a relative. Helping to curb malaria, however, isn't the eucalyptus's only contribution to medicine. The crushed leaves have long been used as an aromatic treatment for respiratory problems. How aromatic? Just faint and find out: Eucalyptus oil is the next best thing to smelling salts.

Therapeutic Uses:
🌿🌿 Asthma, bronchitis, coughing, flu, mucous membrane inflammation, respiratory disease.
🌿 Arthritis, bad breath, cramps, croup, dysentery, fainting, flu, gallbladder problems, infections, muscle pain, ringworm, sinusitis, skin problems, sore throat, worms.

■ Folk uses: Acne, diabetes, fever, gallbladder disease, gum disease, hoarseness, intestinal disease, lack of appetite, liver disease, measles, nerve pain, scarlet fever, sores, whooping cough.

Medicinal Properties:
The pungent vapors of eucalyptus help break up phlegm and bronchial congestion, a welcome action for anyone with bronchitis or a cold. Its cineole is an antiseptic that helps combat bad breath, fight spasms, and kill bacteria and fungi. (It'll make your cheeks rosy, too.) In test tube experiments, eucalyptus's quercetin and hyperoside have been shown to oppose the influenza virus. Its euglobulin helps soothe inflammation.

Prescription Counterparts:
Eucalyptus is the active ingredient in Vicks VapoRub and other decongestants. You'll also find eucalyptol, derived from eucalyptus oil, in over-the-counter cough drops and mouthwashes (check the labels.)

Dosage Options:
Tea made from 1 to 2 teaspoons of chopped dried eucalyptus leaves in a cup of water or ½ to 2 teaspoons of eucalyptus tincture daily. Another alternative is to steep an ounce or so of fresh leaves in about a quart of water, bring the concoction to a boil, and inhale the steam.

Safety Rating: 2

Precautions:
Undiluted, eucalyptus oil is toxic. Less than a teaspoon could be lethal. Signs of an overdose or poisoning include convulsions, delirium, dizziness, gastrointestinal burning, loss of reflexes, and a sense of suffocation. Some people might experience diarrhea or nausea.

EVENING PRIMROSE (Oenothera biennis)

What It Is:
Most flowers like to bask in the sun, but the shiny yellow blossoms of evening primrose (no relation, by the way, to garden primrose) shrink from the sun's rays and bloom at dusk. As the sun rises the next morning, the flowers wilt, and new ones emerge at day's end. Native Americans used all parts of the plant for various teas, tonics, and poultices, and they ate its seeds. Today science recognizes the seed oil as its best source of natural medicine.

Therapeutic Uses:

⚬⚬ Arthritis, breast pain, dementia, diabetic neuropathy, eczema, endometriosis, high blood pressure, osteoporosis, premenstrual tension, prostatitis.

⚬ Alcoholism, Alzheimer's disease, asthma, cancer, colitis, dermatitis, diabetes, heart disease, hardening of the arteries, high cholesterol, hot flashes, hyperactivity, inflammatory bowel disease, itching, kidney disease, liver disease, menstrual irregularities, migraine, multiple sclerosis, Raynaud's disease, schizophrenia, Sjögren's syndrome, skin reddening, stress, stroke, tardive dyskinesia, tissue swelling.

▦ Folk uses: Anxiety, bruises, gastric disease, hair loss, hemorrhoids, indigestion, infertility, muscle inflammation, obesity, psoriasis, whooping cough, wounds.

Medicinal Properties:

Evening primrose's therapeutic value comes courtesy of its rich concentrations of three nutrients. The seed oil contains gamma-linolenic acid (GLA), an omega-6 fatty acid that the body uses to manufacture a prostaglandin vital to soothing inflammation and supporting the immune system. It also helps keep blood flowing freely, reduces high blood pressure, and lowers cholesterol. Research shows that GLA is helpful against arthritis, benign prostatic hypertrophy, eczema, endometriosis, multiple sclerosis, and premenstrual tension, among other conditions. It's also been shown to prevent and reverse the nerve impairment of diabetic neuropathy. Few other plants are such rich sources of GLA (see "Black Currant" on page 41 and "Borage" on page 50). Evening primrose seeds, though not the seeds' oil, are also a good source of the amino acid tryptophan, which the body converts into the mood-improving brain chemical serotonin. The plant's leaves are our best source of a third nutrient, the bioflavonoid quercetin, which keeps blood vessels healthy, improves circulation, and eases asthma.

Dosage Options:

A standardized supplement containing 1,300 milligrams of evening primrose oil and providing at least 130 milligrams of GLA and 960 milligrams of cis-linoleic acid daily. For breast pain, 3 to 4 grams of the oil daily. For eczema, 4 to 8 grams daily. If you're interested in the quercetin, get a standardized supplement of the whole herb rather than the seed oil. You can also eat the leaves, although they're peppery and not very appetizing. (Young leaves are best; mix them with some onion, the second-best source of quercetin.) For tryptophan, much of which is lost in the oil extraction process, take one to five capsules of powdered evening primrose seed.

Safety Rating: 3

Precautions:

None reported. A few hypersensitive people might get a headache or a mild case of nausea. People with schizophrenia who take chlorpromazine (Thorazine) may have difficulty breathing or be at greater risk for epilepsy.

EYEBRIGHT (*Euphrasia*, various species)

What It Is:
The name says it all: Eyebright has always been associated with healthy eyes (or treating unhealthy, inflamed eyes). The species, which grows naturally throughout the northwestern part of North America, boasts almost 200 siblings, all tough to tell apart. They're tiny, no more than about 6 or so inches tall, with small, red-tinged, white flowers that somewhat resemble bloodshot eyes. From the eleventh century on, the plant has been used to treat various eye ailments.

Therapeutic Uses:
▦ Folk uses: Blepharitis (eyelid inflammation), colds, congestion, coughing, hoarseness, nasal membrane disorders, pinkeye, sinusitis, sore throat, styes.

Medicinal Properties:
The long folk medical history and good scientific scrutiny of eyebright notwithstanding, no research has established the plant's value in treating pinkeye and other eye problems. Certain phytochemicals in eyebright display antibacterial, anti-inflammatory, antiseptic, and astringent qualities, but no evidence validates its traditional uses.

Dosage Options:
If you're considering direct application of herbal drops to your eyes, make sure the preparation is sterile. For eyebright eyedrops, consult a doctor who is well-schooled in natural medicine. For ingestion, ½ to 1 teaspoon of a liquid extract daily, ½ to 1 teaspoon of eyebright tincture three times a day, or up to three cups a day of a tea made by steeping 2 to 4 grams of the dried herb in a cup of hot water.

Safety Rating: 1

Precautions:
Over-the-counter eyebright drops may not be sterile. For any solution you plan to put in your eyes, go to an herb-savvy physician. Some research cautions that ingesting 10 to 60 drops of eyebright tincture can cause confusion, constipation, coughing, headache, insomnia, sneezing, and tearing, among other symptoms.

FALSE UNICORN ROOT *(Chamaelirium luteum)*

What It Is:
Native American mothers-to-be munched on the root of this North American plant to deter miscarriage and to treat a variety of problems unique to females. Found principally in moister areas of northeastern North America, but as far south as Florida and as far west as Illinois, false unicorn root may have earned its name from its arching plume of tiny white flowers, which supposedly resembles a unicorn's horn. It's also known as fairy wand, devil's bit, and colicroot.

Therapeutic Uses:
🔎 Infertility, labor, lack of menstruation, menopause, miscarriage, morning sickness.
▦ Folk uses: Colic, fever, indigestion, lack of appetite, liver disease, pain, prostatitis, worms.

Medicinal Properties:
False unicorn root is a time-honored remedy for a whole panoply of uterine and menstrual problems. It may, in fact, help encourage menstruation, but little science backs up its many folk uses. The presence of diosgenin, a hormone precursor, provides a theoretical reason for the folk uses.

Dosage Options:
One-half to 1 teaspoon of a liquid root extract daily, 1 to 2 grams of the root steeped in a cup of hot water and drunk three times a day, or ½ to 1 teaspoon of a root tincture three times a day.

Safety Rating: 1

Precautions:
False unicorn root could irritate your gastrointestinal tract, and excessive amounts could cause nausea or vomiting. Don't take the herb if you're pregnant.

FENNEL *(Foeniculum vulgare)*

What It Is:
This tall, wispy perennial is a staple of both chefs and herbal physicians. Its stems, which have a sweet anise or licorice taste, can be eaten much like celery; its seeds (which are actually one-seeded fruits) spice up recipes for fish and other dishes and contain the most medicinal action. The plant's clusters of tiny yellow flowers resemble upturned umbrellas. Indigenous to the Mediterranean, this member of the parsley family now grows all over the world. A few eastern European countries, Egypt, and China are the major cultivators.

Therapeutic Uses:
🌿🌿 Bronchitis, coughing, gas, gastritis, indigestion, intestinal inflammation, mucous membrane inflammation, respiratory disease.

🌿 Breast milk deficiency, breathing stoppage, colic, constipation, cramps, diarrhea, eye inflammation, hiccups, lack of menstruation, liver disease, low libido, menopause, mouth inflammation, nausea, obesity, pain, stomachache, throat inflammation.

▨ Folk uses: Bed-wetting, cellulite, colitis, heartburn, hernia, inflammatory bowel disease, lack of appetite, prostate cancer, snakebite, vomiting.

Medicinal Properties:
Until 1970, fennel seeds were listed in the U.S. Pharmacopeia. No reason other than America's adoration of synthetic drugs can account for their removal. Fennel is a good digestive aid that relieves gas. Studies show that it quells spasms, facilitates breathing, helps break up chest congestion, and reduces inflammation. Extracts are also estrogenic enough to stimulate the production of breast milk in some women, and a few studies indicate that they perk up the libido of both female and male lab mice.

Prescription Counterparts:
For gas and gastric upset, you might want to test fennel's effectiveness against over-the-counter products such as Mylanta and Gaviscon or against simethicone-containing medications such as Maalox.

Dosage Options:
One-half to 1 teaspoon of a tincture three times a day, 2 to 6 teaspoons of fresh fennel seeds, 1 to 2 teaspoons of mashed fennel seeds stirred into a cup of hot water, ½ ounce or more of fennel syrup, or up to ¼ teaspoon of a liquid seed extract daily.

Safety Rating: 3

Precautions:
Virtually none, particularly when taken as a food (up to 6 grams of seeds per day) or brewed into a tea. Pregnant women and nursing mothers should avoid the essential oil. Isolated cases of allergic asthma reactions have been reported.

FENUGREEK *(Trigonella foenum-graecum)*

What It Is:
Tutankhamen was entombed with seeds from this ancient herb, which has nourished and healed people since the beginning of time. In Egypt, the seeds are baked in breads; in India, they're included in curries; in Africa, they're brewed as a substitute for coffee. You also can eat them by the handful, either cooked or raw. Why bother to eat the seeds at all? Because in ancient Egypt, Greece, and Rome, they were said to be almost a panacea—good for everything from bronchial problems, tuberculosis, and gout to general body pain, swollen glands, skin problems, and low libido. Modern science has uncovered an even more valuable medicinal potential: treating diabetes. Fenugreek originated in southwest Asia and southern Europe, but it's now cultivated in many parts of the world. The plant features oval, minutely serrated leaves, whitish flowers, and seeds that grow inside a pod, much like peas. Coincidentally, fenugreek is a member of the pea family.

Therapeutic Uses:
🖛🖛 Dermatitis, diabetes, high cholesterol, indigestion, inflammation, lack of appetite.

🖛 Arthritis, breast milk deficiency, cancer, constipation, eczema, gas, hair loss, hardening of the arteries, high blood pressure, high triglycerides, infections, labor, sore throat, stone formation in the urinary system, ulcers.

▦ Folk uses: Allergies, boils, bronchitis, coughing, diarrhea, fever, gastritis, gout, hay fever, hernia, intestinal pain, kidney disease, low libido, muscle pain, nerve pain, respiratory disease, sores, stomach disease, swelling, swollen glands, tuberculosis.

Medicinal Properties:
In both laboratory studies on animals and clinical research involving people with type 1 or type 2 diabetes, fenugreek has significantly lowered blood sugar, thanks to some six different phytochemical compounds. That's good news for anyone whose pancreas doesn't secrete enough natural insulin (type 1 diabetes) or anyone whose body tissue just doesn't seem to use insulin efficiently enough to metabolize carbohydrates and sugars (type 2 diabetes). In one study, urinary excretion of glucose plummeted 54 percent after a group of people with type 1 diabetes began to take 50 grams of defatted fenugreek seed powder twice a day. Their fasting blood sugar, low-density lipoprotein (LDL) cholesterol, and blood triglyceride levels also dropped notably. In another experiment involving people with type 2 diabetes, 15 grams of powdered fenugreek seeds markedly lowered after-meal blood sugar readings.

The plant is a decent source of mucilage, a soluble fiber that both absorbs water, thus helping to relieve diarrhea, and softens the stool, thus easing constipation. Mucilage also improves blood cholesterol. In addition, fenugreek contains precursors of phytoestrogens (plant world equivalents of human female hormones), including diosgenin. Chemists often create synthetic estrogens from such materials. Laboratory studies have demonstrated that diosgenin increases milk flow.

According to some anecdotal evidence, it also may help enlarge a woman's breasts and ease menopause-related problems.

Prescription Counterparts:
Although you should not discard your insulin or other medications to regulate blood sugar, you could consider fenugreek. It appears to be at least as safe as, if not quite as effective as, its synthetic prescription counterparts.

Dosage Options:
Studies that have shown fenugreek to be helpful have used extracts of defatted fenugreek seed powder. Specifically, twice-daily dosages were given to people with type 1 (insulin-dependent) diabetes in total daily amounts of 1½ to 2 grams for every 2.2 pounds of body weight. Use only under the guidance of a physician (see "Precautions"). If you don't have diabetes, a typical dosage is 620 milligrams of a standardized extract two or three times a day or a tea made by steeping 1 tablespoon of mashed seeds in a cup of hot water at least once a day. (You can gargle with the tea as well.) You also may eat ¼ to ½ cup of fenugreek seeds, sprouted or unsprouted, every day. For external inflammation or other skin problems, soak 10 teaspoons of powdered seeds in hot water, make a poultice, and apply as often as desired.

Safety Rating: 3

Precautions:
Do not stop taking any diabetes medications that your doctor has prescribed. This herb may or may not work for you. Instead, schedule an appointment with your physician and discuss your interest in fenugreek. Show her the evidence and express your wish to give the herb a try. If you have type 1 diabetes, you may be able to reduce your dosage of and dependence on insulin, which causes weight gain and other problems. If you have type 2 diabetes, you may be able to wean yourself partly off sugar-reducing synthetic medications that raise your risk for heart problems. With repeated external use, some people might experience an allergic reaction. Also, because of fenugreek's fluid-absorbing mucilage, make sure you drink a lot of water.

FEVERFEW 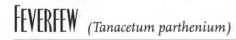 *(Tanacetum parthenium)*

What It Is:
In its traditional use, feverfew, a relative of dandelion and marigolds, supposedly kept fevers at bay. The name is based on *febrifuge,* the scientific term for a fever-reducing medication. Settlers introduced the plant to North America from Europe, and its diminutive daisylike flowers now bloom in the wild and in gardens all over the United States and Canada. Feverfew's leaves exude a powerful, distinctive aroma that freshens the air and reportedly repels bees.

Therapeutic Uses:

∾∾∾ Migraine.

∾ Fever, headache, inflammation, pain.

▦ Folk uses: Allergies, arthritis, asthma, cluster headaches, colds, cramps, dermatitis, dizziness, fever, indigestion, menstrual pain and irregularities, morphine addiction, nausea, neuroses, opium addiction, parasitic infections, stomachache, tinnitus, toothache, worms, wounds.

Medicinal Properties:

Perhaps we should rename this herb "migrainefew." Although laboratory studies have validated its worth in reducing fevers, allergic reactions, and other inflammatory conditions, its best documented use is in preventing and alleviating migraines. A phytochemical called parthenolide most likely is responsible, but don't discount the value of other natural compounds in the plant. Together, they hinder the body's release of inflammatory prostaglandins, deter a process that leads to the thickening or clotting of blood, and tone smooth vascular muscles. Clinical studies have produced mixed results. Some have shown no benefit from feverfew. Others indicate that the herb may be beneficial for as many as two-thirds of all people who have migraines. For instance, according to one British survey of some 300 people who took feverfew daily, 70 percent experienced a reduction in either the frequency or the severity (or both) of their migraines. An Israeli study of 57 migraine sufferers found that feverfew significantly reduced the common symptoms of migraines, including nausea, head pain, and sensitivity to light and noise.

Prescription Counterparts:

Of the 300 or so people cited in the British study, many found no relief from standard migraine medications, which include verapamil (Calan), a calcium channel blocker known to cause side effects such as dizziness, heart rhythm disturbances, nausea, fluid retention, liver problems, and, ironically, headaches. Other scientific studies suggest that feverfew displays qualities (but not side effects) similar to the corticosteroid cortisone and, to a lesser extent, nonsteroidal anti-inflammatory drugs (NSAIDs).

Dosage Options:

Up to 380 milligrams of fresh, powdered leaves as frequently as three times a day or two 25-milligram doses of freeze-dried leaves daily; a teaspoon or two of a liquid leaf extract; or a standardized supplement that contains 250 micrograms of parthenolide daily. Fresh feverfew leaves don't taste all that great, but you might want to try eating up to 4 leaves a day as a preventive. Keep in mind the following precaution though. Feverfew tea tastes somewhat better; steep 2 to 8 leaves in a cup of boiling water to drink at least once a day. (Don't boil the leaves.)

Safety Rating: 2

Precautions:

Not many, if any, for most of us. Chewing on the fresh leaves may cause mouth sores or oral inflammation in some people. Others might experience diarrhea, nausea, flatulence, or vomiting, but usually only during the first week of use. Some sensitive people might notice a mild sedative effect. An extremely remote possibility exists that feverfew could provoke miscarriage.

FLAX *(Linum usitatissimum)*

What It Is:
It's linen. It's linseed oil. It's even in linoleum. It's also just plain old flax, and flax, as its Latin name suggests, is "most useful." The ancient Egyptians spun flax for linen clothing, and fibers have even been found at prehistoric archaeological sites. North American settlers introduced the slim-stemmed, blue-flowered plant to this continent, and it now grows across the northwestern parts of the United States and in Canada. The fibers come from the plant itself; the high-calorie oil, long used to fatten cattle, comes from its seeds. A gummy liquid from the seeds (mucilage) was long used as a poultice to treat burns and other types of inflammation.

Therapeutic Uses:
🐛🐛 Colitis, constipation, diverticulitis, gastritis, high cholesterol, inflammation (general), intestinal inflammation.
🐛 Cancer (especially breast, colon, and endometrial), dermatitis, lupus, kidney disease, mucous membrane inflammation.
▦ Folk uses: Arthritis, boils, bronchitis, burns, colds, coughing, fever, gallbladder problems, gout, lung problems, malaria, mucous membrane inflammation, pleurisy, pneumonia, sore throat, urinary tract infections.

Medicinal Properties:
Two phytochemical compounds give flaxseed its therapeutic edge. The mucilage absorbs water, which softens the stool and encourages better transport through the intestines, making it useful for a variety of gastric complaints. Substances known as lignans help impede the body's use of estrogen, which feeds tumor growth in endometrial and breast cancer. Lignans also may play a role in deterring colon cancer. Flaxseed is one of the best sources of an omega-3 fat called alpha-linolenic acid (ALA), a close chemical cousin of the essential fatty acids in fish oil that have proved so beneficial against everything from inflammation and immune system dysfunction to kidney problems, heart disease, and cancer.

Dosage Options:
One 1,300-milligram capsule standardized for 740 milligrams of ALA daily or 1 tablespoon of whole or crushed seeds two or three times a day.

Safety Rating: 3

Precautions:
Few, if any, reported when taken in reasonable amounts and with sufficient fluid.

The gummy mucilage in flaxseed could cause problems if you have an intestinal obstruction. Abnormally high dosages could upset your body's electrolytes or temporarily cause symptoms of cyanide poisoning. Like any mucilage-containing compound, flaxseed also could interfere with the absorption of medications.

Fo-Ti *(Polygonum multiflorum)*

What It Is:
Part of the knotweed family, this vine's leaves are shaped a little like flat green carrots or even hot peppers. It grows almost everywhere in China, as well as in some American gardens. Practiced healers in traditional Chinese medicine differentiate between the dried, unprocessed root and the cured, processed root, regarding them as entirely different medicinal herbs.

Therapeutic Uses:
🍂🍂 Insomnia, nervous exhaustion, schizophrenia.
🍂 Hardening of the arteries, heart disease, hepatitis, high cholesterol, tumors.
▦ Folk uses: Abscesses, allergies, anemia, athlete's foot, backache, bronchitis, constipation, dermatitis, diabetes, dizziness, enlarged lymph glands, epilepsy, fatigue, graying hair, immune system problems, inflammation, itching, kidney disease, knee pain, nerve inflammation, numbness, ringworm, sores, tinnitus, tuberculosis.

Medicinal Properties:
Processed fo-ti root contains lecithin, which can help deter cholesterol buildup in the liver, the blood, and the interior walls of the arteries. It is also said to combat fatigue and restore the body's vital energy, called *qi*. Unprocessed roots are said to serve as a laxative and blood purifier. In animal studies, fo-ti has shown some ability to encourage the creation of red blood cells, impede bacterial growth, and help acclimate the body to cold weather. Test tube experiments indicate that the emodin in fo-ti can relax blood vessels and modulate the immune system.

Dosage Options:
Two or three 560-milligram capsules of a standardized extract three times a day or ½ to 1 dropper of a concentrated liquid root extract two or three times a day. You can also steep 3 to 5 grams of dried fo-ti in a cup of hot water and drink three times a day.

Safety Rating: 3

Precautions:
Few reported. For some very sensitive people, raw fo-ti could cause vomiting; the processed root could cause gastric upset and aggravate diarrhea. Some people might notice numbness or tingling in their arms or legs.

FOXGLOVE, CHINESE *(Rehmannia glutinos)*

See "Rehmannia" on page 184.

GARCINIA *(Garcinia cambogia)*

See "Malabar Tamarind" on page 145.

GARLIC *(Allium sativum)*

What It Is:

If garlic didn't exist, the great pyramids might not exist. The pungent bulb supposedly imbued Egyptians with the strength to erect those mammoth structures. And without garlic, the world would have been overcome by vampires long ago. The plant, which has long, flat, pointy leaves and pinkish white flowers, is native to Europe but now grows naturally in the central United States. It also thrives in Gilroy, California, the "Garlic Capital of the World," and in any garden that enjoys a lot of warm, sunny weather.

A cousin of onion, leek, chive, and shallot, and a more distant kin of lily and aloe, garlic has been employed since ancient times as both food and medicine. People have used it to treat colds and sore throats, ease intestinal discomfort, take the kink out of rheumatic complaints, and fight off viruses and other infectious marauders. Given the bulb's blow to that "ol' factory" in your nose, some herbal authorities theorize that it worked in the past simply because it maintained a good arm's length or two between the wearer and everybody else. We now know better. Garlic is potent medicine, arguably one of the best that nature has to offer.

Therapeutic Uses:

〰〰〰 Athlete's foot, hardening of the arteries, heart disease, high cholesterol, high triglycerides, intermittent claudication, Raynaud's disease.

〰〰 Bedsores, bronchitis, burns, cancer, colds, coughing, diarrhea, dysentery, fever, gastroenteritis, intestinal disease, liver poisoning from acetaminophen, high blood pressure, immune system problems, oral inflammation, pharyngitis, vaginitis, warts and other bumpy skin growths, whooping cough, yeast infections.

〰 Abscesses, Alzheimer's disease, appendicitis, arthritis, asthma, bronchiectasis (dilation of the lungs' bronchial tubes, characterized by terribly bad breath, a cough, and pus-filled expectoration), cholera, colic, colitis, cytomegalovirus, diabetes, earache, ear inflammation, flu, fungal infections, gas, gum disease, hair loss, herpes, HIV, hookworm, indigestion, kidney disease, laryngitis, lead poisoning, liver disease, mouth ulcers, mucous membrane swelling, nausea, nerve pain, nicotine addiction, pneumonia, respiratory disease, ringworm, roundworm, skin problems, sores, sore throat, stroke (ischemic), tuberculosis, typhus, viral infections (including poliomyelitis), worms.

▦ Folk uses: Acne, convulsions, corns, diarrhea, gallbladder problems, gout, lupus, menstrual irregularities, muscle pain, sciatica, skin problems, snakebite, tissue swelling, water retention, wounds.

Medicinal Properties:

Allicin is the most often-cited phytomedicinal in garlic, but the bulb actually contains some 70 active ingredients with a broad range of therapeutic capabilities that have been explored and demonstrated in more than 2,000 studies. The stinky herb is probably our premier plant for virtually any heart or circulatory condition. It lowers blood pressure (the systolic reading by 20 to 30 points and the diastolic reading by 10 to 20 points, according to some studies done on people with hypertension). It cuts low-density lipoprotein (LDL) cholesterol by some 10 to 12 percent and triglycerides by about 15 percent, and it markedly impedes LDL's oxidation into artery-clogging atherosclerotic plaque. Nine separate substances also thin the blood and deter its tendency to clot.

Garlic lowers the incidence of cancer, particularly in the gastrointestinal system (allicin interferes with the creation of carcinogenic nitrosamines in the stomach) and fortifies the body's natural defenses, notably by doubling the activity of natural killer cells in the bloodstream. As first noted by the nineteenth-century scientist Louis Pasteur, garlic juice kills a variety of bacteria. We now know that allicin and other sulfur compounds also destroy many parasites, fungi, and viruses, including *Helicobacter pylori* (which causes peptic ulcers), staphylococcus, streptococcus, E. coli, salmonella, *Candida albicans*, herpes, and influenza.

Prescription Counterparts:

Garlic doesn't only fend off folkloric bloodsuckers; it can ward off the pharmaceutical industry's vampires, too. The bulb's cholesterol-lowering ability compares very favorably with such highly touted drugs as simvastatin (Zocor) and atorvastatin (Lipitor). Both medications can cause liver problems and loss of libido. (Garlic, by contrast, might gently boost libido, thanks to the presence of free arginine, an amino acid.) Zocor might cause muscle cramps or pain, dizziness, tremors, eye problems, anxiety, and skin eruptions, among other side effects. Lipitor could inflict facial swelling, fever, gastric upset, oral irritation, urinary problems, sleepiness, and leg cramps.

The bulb opposes fungal infections better than a handful of other noted fungus killers, including nystatin (Mycostatin). And it compares favorably to drugs such as penicillin, erythromycin, and tetracycline, counteracting bacterial infections that prescription antibiotics may no longer touch. Bacteria are smart; they quickly develop a resistance to the single-minded focus of pharmaceutical antibiotics. But they're less able to defend themselves against the multifaceted "shotgun" attack of garlic's phytochemicals. The bulb enhances the action of prescription antibiotics as well.

In fact, garlic intensifies the action of a number of pharmaceuticals. Some interpret that as an argument against ingesting the bulb therapeutically (see "Precautions"). However, you should more optimistically consider it an indication of the herb's potential to lessen your reliance on costly medications that have potentially perilous side effects.

Use garlic only in conjunction with your physician, not on your own. Ideally, you'll be able to locate an herb-savvy doctor who knows what to do. If you cannot, tell your regular doctor about your intention to try a more natural approach and ask that he monitor your progress carefully.

Dosage Options:

Garlic is the finest in "food farmacy." You don't need extracts or isolated compounds for a medicinal effect; you can ingest the whole herb. As a matter of fact, the whole herb likely is better than any processed supplement out there. Try eating 1 to 5 cloves every day. Or take ½ to 1 teaspoon of garlic juice or ½ to 2 teaspoons of garlic syrup daily.

This aromatic healer also works topically. For athlete's foot, crush a couple of cloves in a basin, add some warm water and a little alcohol, and soak your feet. To treat vaginitis, create a homemade tampon-like package by peeling a whole garlic clove without nicking it, wrapping it in sterile gauze, and securing it with clean, unbleached string.

If you want to take garlic supplementally, try taking one 400-milligram capsule or tablet standardized to contain at least 3 milligrams of allicin every day. Eschew supplements that supposedly leave you odor-free. Allicin gives cut or crushed garlic its distinctive aroma and much of its medicinal strength. When you cut or crush garlic, you release the allicin, and it begins to dissipate. Marketers of deodorized garlic supplements may disagree, but the smell is part of getting well: The more it stinks, the more good it does.

Safety Rating: 3

Precautions:
Virtually none when taken in rational therapeutic amounts. You'll no doubt have a garlicky scent on your breath and perhaps your skin. Some unusually sensitive people might experience an allergic skin reaction or suffer an asthma attack (even upon inhalation of garlic powder from the spice rack). Others might become nauseous or get diarrhea. If you consume more than five cloves a day, you could get heartburn or notice some flatulence. Massive doses might cause dizziness, bloating, headache, or profuse sweating. As with other piquant plants, direct application might irritate your skin.

As mentioned, garlic complements the effects of many prescription drugs—drugs on which you might reduce your dependence if you work closely with an herb-friendly physician. Such medications include nonsteroidal anti-inflammatory drugs (NSAIDs), anticoagulants, cimetidine (Tagamet), ciprofloxacin (Cipro), clarithromycin (Biaxin), diltiazem (Cardizem), enoxacin (Penetrex), erythromycin, fluoxetine (Prozac), fluvoxamine (Luvox), itraconazole (Sporanox), ketoconazole (Nizoral), nefazodone (Serzone), paroxetine (Paxil), and ritonavir (Norvir). Garlic also may interact with and magnify the effectiveness of drugs metabolized by the liver, including alprazolam (Xanax), amitriptyline (Elavil), astemizole (Hismanal), carbamazepine (Tegretol), cisapride (Propulsid), clozapine (Clozaril), corticosteroids, cyclosporine (Neoral), Desipramine, diazepam (Valium), imipramine (Tofranil), and phenytoin (Coumadin).

GENTIAN *(Gentiana lutea)*

What It Is:
This handsome ornamental herb has large clusters of big, orange yellow flowers and stiff, pointy, yellow green leaves that resemble those on lady's slipper. The roots have been used since the first century as a bitter tonic to improve digestion. In medieval Europe, they were considered a poison antidote. In the mid-1800s, they were popularly mixed with licorice and billed as a patent medicine to curb tobacco use. The remedy may or may not work, and both gentian and licorice have their own minor side effects, although those complications pale in comparison to the impact of tobacco.

Therapeutic Uses:
⚕⚕ Gas, indigestion, lack of appetite.
⚕ Gastritis, heartburn, stomachache, stomach disease, tobacco addiction, ulcers, wounds.

▦ Folk uses: Arthritis, bronchitis, diarrhea, jaundice, nausea, sore throat.

Medicinal Properties:
Gentian roots' bitterness increases gastric secretions and makes your mouth water—for something to kill its nasty taste. Perhaps that's why they are widely used in Europe as an appetite stimulant. Gentian also promotes digestion and calms an upset stomach.

Dosage Options:
One teaspoon of powdered gentian root in 3 cups of water, 20 to 40 drops of gentian tincture, ½ to 1 teaspoon of a liquid extract, or ½ to 1 teaspoon of fresh roots daily.

Safety Rating: 1

Precautions:
Certain compounds in gentian, including gentisin and isogentisin, reportedly can cause genetic mutations, so use of the root probably should be avoided if you're pregnant or nursing. In addition, the root, especially if used to excess, could generate too much gastric acid and upset your stomach.

GERMAN CHAMOMILE *(Matricaria recutita)*

See "Chamomile, German" on page 69.

GINGER *(Zingiber officinale)*

What It Is:
The thick, knotty rhizome of this perennial plant has been a culinary and medicinal mainstay for thousands of years. Probably half of the herbal formulas in traditional Chinese medicine include ginger as an active ingredient, usually to soothe the stomach, encourage appetite, and offset the effects of other strong natural medicines. Native to Asia, ginger is now grown in a number of tropical countries, including India, Nigeria, and Haiti. Jamaica is the world's leading cultivator. The common name comes from a Sanskrit word meaning "horn-shaped"; the botanical name is from the Greek word for the root, *zingiberis*.

Therapeutic Uses:
🍃🍃 Dizziness, indigestion, lack of appetite, morning sickness, motion sickness, postoperative nausea, seasickness.
🍃 Alcoholism, arthritis, backache, blood clots, burns, chemotherapy-related nausea, colds, colic, coughing, cramps, depression, diarrhea, flu, gas, gastritis,

headache, heart disease, inflammation, intestinal disease, liver disease, low libido, lumbago, menstrual irregularities, migraine, muscle pain, nausea, sore throat, stroke, tissue swelling, ulcers, water retention.

※ Folk uses: Aging, cataracts, dandruff, earache, fever, hair loss, hardening of the arteries, hemorrhoids, insomnia, kidney disease, toothache.

Medicinal Properties:

Ginger's well-documented, world-renowned digestive and intestinal relief comes courtesy of a number of phytochemicals. Its gingerols and shogaols quell stomach upset and gently but effectively encourage the muscle contractions that move food through your intestines. At the same time, oddly enough, they inhibit spasms, curb diarrhea, and deter the urge to vomit. The root's oleoresins, proteolytic enzymes, and essential oils also improve the movement of food through the gastrointestinal tract, and they neutralize stomach acids and digestive toxins. The overall impact off-sets the effects of excessive motion, overindulgence, and improper chewing. Taking 1 gram of powdered ginger (about ½ teaspoon) quelled vomiting, dizziness, and cold sweats in a group of U.S. Navy cadets who had yet to develop their sea legs. Other research demonstrates that ginger lessens chemotherapy-induced nausea; morning sickness and pregnancy-related vomiting; and, at least in animals, gastric ulcers, particularly those caused by indomethacin and aspirin, as well as by ethanol.

Zingibain and other phytochemical compounds in ginger quench inflammation. Zingibain is a proteolytic enzyme that breaks down proteins (much like meat ten-derizers) and counteracts inflammation, inhibiting certain prostaglandins and other inflammation-igniting, pain-causing, tissue-swelling substances. In a 2-year Indian experiment, 36 of 48 people with rheumatoid arthritis or osteoarthritis enjoyed at least some abatement of joint pain (and absolutely no side effects) after taking 3 to 7 grams of fresh ginger daily. In another test of the herb's therapeutic value, 56 people with rheumatoid arthritis, osteoarthritis, or fibromyalgia ingested 2 to 4 teaspoons of powdered ginger daily. More than 75 percent of the study's par-ticipants ended up notably free of pain. (In case you were wondering, just 1 gram of zingibain will tenderize up to 20 pounds of meat. It's one of nature's best prote-olytic enzymes. Some experts say that it's at least as effective as the papain in papaya and the bromelain in pineapple. For more information, see "Papaya" on page 163 and "Pineapple" on page 173.)

Ginger also offers a number of antioxidant compounds that help keep blood fats from forming arterial plaque. Perhaps better than garlic and onion, it inhibits sub-stances that thicken the blood and encourage blood clotting. And by stimulating the secretion of bile and hindering fat absorption, ginger improves cholesterol levels.

Prescription Counterparts:

Ginger poses a major threat to certain segments of the pharmaceutical industry, as illustrated in several head-to-head comparisons. In one study, 940 milligrams of powdered root alleviated the wooziness of motion sickness better than 100 mil-ligrams of the antihistamine dimenhydrinate. For postsurgical nausea and vomit-ing, ginger equaled the effectiveness of metoclopramide, a drug whose long list of side effects includes confusion, depression, drowsiness or insomnia, diarrhea, visual disturbances, and the emergence of involuntary (possibly irreversible) jerky or parkinsonian movements. Other research has established that ginger works just as well as stomach-irritating, ulcer-inducing aspirin at reducing swelling and water retention, as well as preventing blood clotting. The herb's gingerols are stronger inhibitors of inflammatory prostaglandins than indomethacin.

Dosage Options:
One 480-milligram standardized supplement twice a day, 2 teaspoons of powdered root in a cup of hot water daily, 3 to 10 grams of fresh ginger or 2 to 4 grams of dried ginger up to three times a day, up to ½ teaspoon of a liquid extract daily, or ½ to 1 teaspoon of ginger tincture or ginger syrup every day. Soak a towel in some ginger tea and apply it directly to the skin to ease a headache, joint stiffness, or abdominal cramps. You can, of course, also drink ginger ale. Just make sure it contains real ginger and is not artificially flavored. (Some manufacturers still use the real thing.)

Safety Rating: 3

Precautions:
If you take an excessively large amount of ginger (say, more than 6 grams) on an empty stomach, it might irritate your gastrointestinal tract. Otherwise, ginger is supremely safe. The herb could magnify the effects of prescription blood thinners and could intensify the impaired blood-clotting ability often seen in chemotherapy. For a few people, ginger might cause heartburn. People with gallstones probably should talk to an herbal expert before ingesting the root therapeutically.

GINKGO *(Ginkgo biloba)*

What It Is:
When *Tyrannosaurus rex* roamed the earth and pterodactyls ruled the sky, there was ginkgo. It's the oldest tree species in the world, and because it's almost indestructible—virtually invulnerable to disease, bugs, and pollution—each tree can live more than a thousand years. The deciduous ginkgo may grow 100 feet or more tall, with fanlike, Y-shaped leaves and yellow green fruits that resemble plums—at least in size and shape. In terms of aroma, they're repugnantly fetid, smelling somewhat like rancid butter. The Chinese began taking ginkgo several thousand years ago to ward off age-related mental decline. Science has belatedly validated that use, along with other medicinal applications.

Therapeutic Uses:
🌿🌿 Altitude sickness, Alzheimer's disease, blood flow deficiency to the brain, dizziness, intermittent claudication, macular degeneration, menstrual irregularities, oxygen deficiency to tissue (hypoxia), senility, sexual dysfunction, tinnitus.

🍂 Allergies, anxiety, arthritis, asthma, blood constriction or clotting, bronchitis, capillary fragility, cellulite, circulatory deficiency, depression, dizziness, emphysema, excessive thirst (as from uncontrolled diabetes), eye inflammation, fatigue, hair loss, hardening of the arteries, headache, hearing loss, heart disease, labor, migraine, nerve pain, premenstrual tension, Raynaud's disease, retinal disease and inflammation, scabies, shock, sores, stroke, tissue swelling, tuberculosis, vaginal disease, varicose veins, water retention, worms.

▨ Folk uses: Chilblains, coughing, dermatitis, diabetes, diarrhea, freckles, multiple sclerosis, nasal inflammation, urinary excess (as from diabetes), vaginal infections, worms.

Medicinal Properties:

Hundreds of clinical and animal experiments, most of them conducted in Europe, have established the therapeutic value of ginkgo's phytochemicals. The bilobalides, ginkgolides, flavonoids, and other substances unique to the tree restore better blood flow to all parts of the body but particularly to the brain, allowing improved use of oxygen. They also stabilize the structure of brain and nerve cells and protect them from oxidative attacks by free radicals. The net result is that you remain more cerebrally supple, able to forestall the memory loss, lack of mental dexterity, and depressive tendencies that so often accompany aging.

What works for the brain works for the rest of you, too. Protecting cells, thinning the blood, and warding off blood vessel blockages maintain healthier circulation in your arms, legs, and eyes. The research demonstrates that ginkgo extracts help prevent or relieve intermittent claudication, Raynaud's disease, and other types of peripheral vascular insufficiency; macular degeneration and, at least in rats, diabetic retinopathy; circulation-related tinnitus and loss of hearing; and sexual dysfunction from lack of genital blood flow. After taking 60 to 120 milligrams of a ginkgo extract twice a day, 91 percent of 33 women and 76 percent of 30 men reported a higher libido, improved erection and lubrication, and better orgasms.

Allergies and asthma also improve with ginkgo. The herb contains a dozen different anti-inflammatory chemicals and seven natural antihistamines. The ginkgolides also interfere with the body's release of a protein that provokes asthmatic bronchial spasms.

Prescription Counterparts:

No pharmaceutical equivalent exists for improving cerebral circulation. Mainstream American medicine offers nothing for this common consequence of aging. For Alzheimer's disease, the pharmaceutical industry provides tacrine (Cognex), a drug known to cause nausea, vomiting, and increased risk of ulcers and liver problems, including jaundice.

Against the activity-induced leg pain of intermittent claudication, ginkgo is the herbal treatment of choice. It outperforms by far doctors' chosen prescription treatment, pentoxiphylline (Trental), enabling people to walk much farther before discomfort sets in. The herb bested the pharmaceutical in nine double-blind studies. The studies show that Trental, which improves blood flow by reducing its viscosity, lengthens pain-free walking distance by about 65 percent. In the process, however, it also can cause nausea, bloating, flatulence, dizziness, and headaches. Ginkgo, by contrast, lengthens pain-free walking distance by some 300 percent. It has few, if any, side effects, and it costs less than half as much as the pharmaceutical. (The best treatment for intermittent claudication, though, remains regular exercise.)

In the erectile dysfunction experiment cited in "Medicinal Properties," none of the men had been helped by one of medicine's standard treatments, penile injections of papaverine, a vasodilator and smooth-muscle relaxant. For those who did not improve after taking ginkgo, the herb at least enabled some of them to respond better to the drug. Since this study was performed, science has given us sildenafil citrate (Viagra), which may work better than ginkgo but may not be as safe in the long run.

Ginkgo extracts also improved hearing loss of unknown origin just as well as (and with far fewer side effects than) a pharmaceutical and minimized salicylate-induced tinnitus and hearing loss.

Dosage Options:
One 40-milligram capsule standardized to contain at least 24 percent flavonoid glycosides three times a day; ⅛ teaspoon of a liquid extract three times a day; 1 to 2 tablespoons of fresh ginkgo leaves every day; or ⅛ teaspoon of ginkgo tincture three times a day. The longer you take ginkgo, the more apparent its benefits become.

Safety Rating: 2

Precautions:
Although many herbalists consider ginkgo to be poisonous, side effects from supplemental extracts are rare and mild, if they occur at all. Some people might experience diarrhea, a skin reaction, an upset stomach, headaches, or insomnia. The bilobetin and ginkgolic acid in the tree are similar to the irritating phytochemical in poison ivy. Handling the leaves can provoke a skin reaction, as can touching the pulp of the fruit. Consuming too many of the seeds can be toxic—even lethal. Avoid ginkgo if you're taking monoamine oxidase inhibitors (MAOIs) for depression.

Sudden nosebleeds or bleeding gums could be a sign that you're taking too much ginkgo. Because the herb thins the blood, you should be especially careful if you have hemophilia or another clotting disorder. The same holds true if you're taking prescription blood thinners; ginkgo enhances the therapeutic impact of such drugs.

This note isn't so much a warning as it is a word to the wise: If you want to lessen your reliance on potentially dangerous drugs and, in the process, save a lot of money, ask your doctor to modify your drug dosages based on how ginkgo helps normalize your vascular health.

GINSENG, ORIENTAL (Panax ginseng)

What It Is:

Ginseng is arguably the best-known and one of the most extensively prescribed herbs in Chinese medicine, used as a general adaptogenic and restorative tonic for just about any problem. Several of a dozen or more species of *Panax* are used medicinally or culinarily: oriental ginseng (also called Chinese or Korean ginseng and the subject of this entry), American ginseng *(P. quinquefolius)*, Japanese ginseng *(P. pseudoginseng Japonicum)*, Himalayan ginseng *(P. pseudoginseng)*, Tienchi ginseng *(P. pseudoginseng Notoginseng)*, and dwarf ginseng *(P. trifolium)*. Of late, a few scientists have looked at Vietnamese ginseng *(P. vietnamensis)*. Some tout Siberian ginseng *(Eleutherococcus senticosus)*. Although it shares some of the same chemical constituents, it's from a different genus in the Aralia family. Other species of the genus *Eleutherococcus* also are used medicinally and ornamentally.

The many ginseng species are commonly confused and sometimes used interchangeably in supplements. Remember that this entry applies only to oriental ginseng *(P. ginseng)*, the best studied of the bunch. (Curiously, although people who live in Asia regard oriental ginseng most favorably, they also are the best customers of American ginseng.) Oriental ginseng usually features five-fingered leaves and green white flowers that are followed by bright red berries. But the true health-promoting value is underground in the roots, which sometimes take the shape of an abstract human form. They contain many of the active phytochemicals and gave rise to the original Chinese name for the plant, *jen shen,* which means "man root."

Therapeutic Uses:

🍂🍂 Exhaustion, fatigue, infirmity, liver disease, stress, wasting from chronic disease, weakness.

🍂 Alcoholism, Alzheimer's disease, cancer, diabetes (types 1 and 2), gastritis, high cholesterol, immune system problems, infertility, liver cancer, lung cancer, low libido, radiation sickness, shock, ulcers.

▦ Folk uses: Amnesia, anxiety, arthritis, asthma, breathing difficulties, chest pain, colds, colitis, convulsions, coughing, depression, fever, headache, heart disease, hypothermia, indigestion, infections, irregular heart rhythm, lack of appetite, menopause, mental derangement, morning sickness, nerve pain, neuroses, palpitations, prolapse, tuberculosis.

Medicinal Properties:

A baker's dozen of ginsenosides, along with other compounds, may explain the roots' wide-ranging therapeutic properties. Either individually or collectively, the phytomedicines have been shown to both sharpen performance and alertness and slow reaction time, heighten sensitivity to stress and deaden feelings of anxiety, and reduce high blood pressure and elevate low blood pressure. Some herbal authorities argue that producing these seemingly contradictory effects is precisely what an adaptogen is supposed to do: balance out body chemistry no matter what the disparity. Many American scientists aren't convinced, but clinical studies involving people and animals, as well as test tube experiments, suggest that ginseng may boost mood, improve memory and attention, lengthen physical and mental endurance, improve test scores, and ease anxiety. It also might help balance blood fats, normalize blood pressure, stabilize blood sugar, rev up several immune system components, ward off colds and other infections, reduce the risk of cancer, buck up the liver in filtering out toxins and synthesizing protein, support normal sexual development, increase sexual activity, counteract some symptoms of menopause, and restore more normal function to the thyroid and adrenal glands.

Dosage Options:
One or two 250-milligram capsules standardized for 5 to 9 percent ginsenosides, 1 tablespoon of fresh roots, or ¼ to a little more than 1 teaspoon of a liquid extract daily, or ½ teaspoon of dried root in a cup of hot water up to twice a day.

Safety Rating: 3

Precautions:
Few recorded when used in reasonable amounts. Some very sensitive people might get an upset stomach, and some women might notice a little breast pain or tenderness or some menstrual irregularity. Chronic use might cause headaches. High doses might cause diarrhea, insomnia, nervous irritability, euphoria, tremors, palpitations, or skin reactions. Large amounts also might raise blood pressure or impair sexual function. Pregnant women, nursing mothers, and babies should not take ginseng. A few observers caution that you shouldn't take ginseng with coffee or other stimulants or if you have a heart problem. Some herbal experts attribute reported side effects to the use of low-quality, adulterated preparations.

GOLDENROD (Solidago virgaurea)

What It Is:
When early American tax protesters tossed all that tea into Boston Harbor, the colonists turned to, among other plants, goldenrod, brewing its long, thin leaves into what was called liberty tea. They were using socially what Native Americans had long used medicinally. Americans took advantage of some of the 20 or so native species of this tall, aromatic perennial, which in the fall is topped with bright yellow flowers. But the species discussed here, *S. virgaurea,* wasn't one of them. It's a native of Europe, where it was a favored treatment for water retention, urinary complaints, and intestinal problems.

Therapeutic Uses:
🌿🌿 Bladder stones, inflammation, kidney stones, urinary tract infections, water retention.

🐦 Kidney inflammation, oral inflammation, pharyngitis, wounds.

▦ Folk uses: Arthritis, diabetes, eczema, gout, hemorrhoids, infections, tuberculosis.

Medicinal Properties:
Goldenrod is a decent diuretic, making it useful for various urinary complaints and water retention. Its phytochemicals also display some anti-inflammatory, pain-relieving, and immune-stimulating qualities.

Dosage Options:
Six to 15 grams of the chopped dried herb in a cup of boiling water or ½ to 1 teaspoon of a liquid leaf extract daily.

Safety Rating: 2

Precautions:
None reported. People with chronic kidney disease or another serious kidney condition should talk to a physician before taking goldenrod.

GOLDENSEAL *(Hydrastis canadensis)*

What It Is:
To Native Americans and newcomers to the continent, goldenseal was a folk medicine staple, a surefire, infection-fighting antibiotic and antiseptic that also stopped bleeding and hemorrhaging. The low plant, which grows naturally only in shaded forests across the eastern and central part of the United States, bears just one green white flower, which is followed by a raspberry-like fruit. You'll have to dig deeper for the natural medicine, though, for the bright yellow roots contain the active ingredients and also produce a nice dye.

Therapeutic Uses:
🐦 Bronchitis, canker sores, cholera, colds, colitis, cramps, Crohn's disease, dermatitis, diabetes (type 2), diarrhea, dysentery, earache, ear discharge, ear inflammation, eczema, eye diseases (specifically, contagious ones such as trachoma, which can lead to blindness), eye inflammation, gallbladder problems, gastritis, gingivitis, gonorrhea, heart disease, herpes, indigestion, infections, irregular heart rhythm, jaundice, kidney inflammation, lack of appetite, laryngitis, menstrual irregularities (including excessive menstrual flow), oral inflammation, parasitic infections (including giardiasis, leishmaniasis, ringworm, salmonella, and tapeworm), pharyngitis, pneumonia, smallpox, sores, trichomoniasis, tuberculosis, ulcers, urinary tract infections, vaginitis.

▦ Folk uses: Acne, alcohol addiction, asthma, cancer, chafing, congestion, constipation, coughing, dandruff, flu, hemorrhage, hemorrhoids, muscle pain, sciatica, sore throat, tinnitus, uterine bleeding, vaginal discharge.

Medicinal Properties:
Berberine and hydrastine give goldenseal its broad-spectrum antibiotic, antiseptic, antifungal, antiparasitic, antiviral, and all-around antimicrobial might. (Barberry, goldthread, Oregon grape, and yellowroot also contain berberine.) Other substances, including berberastine and hydrastinine, play supporting roles. Berberine triggers white blood cells to seek out bacteria, viruses, fungi, and even tumor cells. (Some research suggests that it kills tumor cells directly.) It also stimulates more blood flow to the spleen, which filters the blood and generates immune-activating substances. And even in amounts that don't directly kill the bug, berberine prevents streptococci from latching onto our cells, thus preventing a common infection without posing the threat that the bacteria will build up an immunity to the treatment.

Prescription Counterparts:
In research featuring head-to-head matchups between pharmaceuticals and goldenseal, the plant performed at least as well, if not better, especially against infectious diarrhea and other gastrointestinal bugs. For instance, in a study of children infected by giardia, goldenseal bested the pharmaceutical metronidazole (Flagyl), eliminating symptoms for 48 percent of the kids after 6 days, compared with 33 percent for the drug. In a study involving 200 adults with diarrhea, berberine added to conventional antibiotic treatment sped healing over antibiotic treatment alone.

According to another experiment, the berberine in goldenseal was more active than the prescription antibiotic chloramphenicol (Chloromycetin) in treating stye-causing staph infections. And in a comparative study against the drug sulfacetamide (Sultrin), the mainstream treatment of choice for vision-impairing trachoma infections, berberine took longer to work but did the job far more thoroughly. Sulfacetamide minimized symptoms sooner but allowed a lot of relapses because the drug did not eradicate the bug from the participants' bodies. Berberine eased symptoms, too, and also eliminated *Chlamydia trachomatis* in every person; none of them suffered a recurrence of symptoms.

Dosage Options:
For a standardized supplement, 465 milligrams two or three times a day; for dried or powdered forms of the whole herb, 535 to 1,075 milligrams three times a day. Other options include ¼ teaspoon of a liquid root extract once a day, 1 dropper of goldenseal tincture three times a day, or ½ to 1 teaspoon of the powdered root in hot water daily. To treat canker sores, let the tea cool and use it as a mouth rinse three or four times a day.

Safety Rating: 1

Precautions:
Goldenseal is not for long-term use; consult a qualified physician. Large doses of the supplement or use of the fresh plant might irritate the mouth and throat or cause diarrhea or vomiting. Big doses of hydrastine could raise blood pressure, induce convulsions, cause exaggerated reflexes, and, in the most extreme cases, lead to respiratory failure and death.

GOTU KOLA *(Centella asiatica)*

What It Is:

Don't assume anything simply from the name of this low-lying herb, which sports umbrella-like leaves on stalks ascending from creeping stems that hug the earth. It is not related to the cola nut of the chocolate family. Gotu kola, which grows in tropical Africa, America, Asia, and Australia, is part of the parsley family. Any go-to-it restorative effect it imparts does not come from caffeine. An ancient Ayurvedic medicine also dispensed in China, Australia, Indonesia, the South Pacific, and southern Africa, gotu kola is used topically and internally to rejuvenate and perpetuate both brain and body. As herbal observers noted in ages gone by, elephants like to eat gotu kola's semicircular leaves. We all know that elephants live long and never forget. Science has since suggested that those elephants might be on the right track: Experiments show that the plant does improve memory.

Therapeutic Uses:

🖛🖛 Arthritis, bedsores, burns, chronic venous insufficiency, keloids, scleroderma, sores, stretch marks, ulcers, wounds.

🖛 Arthritis, cellulite, cholera, cirrhosis, hair loss, hemorrhoids, hepatitis, kidney inflammation, leprosy, memory failure, psoriasis, scars, tissue swelling, varicose veins, water retention.

▦ Folk uses: Anemia, asthma, boils, bronchitis, bruises, constipation, dementia, diarrhea, dizziness, dysentery, eczema, elephantiasis, epilepsy, fever, fractures, headache, high blood pressure, jaundice, lupus, measles, menstrual irregularities, neuroses, nosebleeds, phlebitis, schizophrenia, scleroderma, skin problems, smallpox, sprains, stomachache, tuberculosis, urinary pain or problems, vomiting of blood.

Medicinal Properties:

Clinical studies over the years have proved that gotu kola is a good skin and tissue rejuvenator. It speeds healing of wounds of all kinds (including burns, ulcers, and surgical incisions) and deters scarring and keloid formation. One small study even offered hope for people with the connective tissue disease scleroderma. After taking just 20 milligrams of an extract three times a week, only 2 of 13 study participants failed to experience better finger dexterity, less joint pain, and a reduction in skin hardness.

People with varicose veins and other vein-related disorders benefit, too. Lack of sufficient blood flow, leg swelling, leg cramps, spider veins, numbness, and a heavy feeling in the legs all improved for about 80 percent of the people who ingested extracts as part of clinical studies. Other studies have demonstrated that the herb even helps reduce cellulite and deters a far greater skin affliction: leprosy.

Scientists don't know precisely how or why gotu kola heals and regenerates body tissue, but they're setting their sights on phytochemicals such as asiaticoside, asiatic acid, and other triterpenes. These substances appear to support connective tissue and blood vessels, maintain the structural integrity of the protective sheaths that surround our veins, and buck up the body's production of such connective building blocks as chondroitin sulfate and hyaluronic acid. In animal experiments, asiaticoside even accelerated the growth of hair and nails.

Prescription Counterparts:
Clinical studies show that gotu kola works just about as well as the antileprosy drug dapsone.

Dosage Options:
Sixty to 120 milligrams of a supplement standardized for triterpenoids daily, ½ to 1 teaspoon of a liquid extract daily, 1 to 2 teaspoons of the dried herb in a cup of hot water three times a day, 2 to 4 teaspoons of a tincture three times a day, or ¼ cup of fresh leaves daily.

Safety Rating: 2

Precautions:
A few people might notice some itchiness or other skin reactions; others might become temporarily oversensitive to sunlight. Some research hints that repeated topical exposure to the asiaticoside in gotu kola could cause skin cancer. Be cautious if you're taking prescription drugs for depression, high blood pressure, or high cholesterol. Extremely large doses might induce nausea.

GRAPE; GRAPE SEED *(Vitis vinifera)*

What It Is:
Don't eat seedless grapes. If you do, you'll deprive yourself of some of the natural medicine in this healthful plant. Grapes were first stomped into wine some 5,000 years ago in Egypt, and they've been used therapeutically ever since. The astringent leaves were used to heal such wide-ranging complaints as diarrhea and varicose veins. The unripened fruit was said to soothe sore throats, while the dried fruit (otherwise known as the raisin) helped not only sore throats but also coughs. Only in the past few decades, though, has science begun to unlock the secrets of the seeds.

Therapeutic Uses:
Anaphylactic shock, arthritis, cancer, capillary fragility, caries, gout, hardening of the arteries, heart disease, hepatitis, high cholesterol, HIV, infections, inflammation, macular degeneration, night blindness, retinopathy, stomach disease, sunburn, tissue swelling, ulcers, varicose veins, water retention, wounds, wrinkles.

Medicinal Properties:
Like grape seeds, wine and whole grapes have a host of phytomedicinal compounds that relieve pain, reduce inflammation, and protect the cardiovascular system from

free radical harm. Among them are a group of flavonoids called oligomeric pro-cyanidins (OPCs). Found abundantly in an extract of grape seeds (pine bark and peanut husks are other sources), OPCs possess a dramatic ability to protect and tone capillaries, with reportedly some 50 times more antioxidant might than even vitamins C and E. Studies suggest that their therapeutic potential comes into play against a number of microcirculatory problems, from chronic venous insufficiency and varicose veins to macular degeneration and diabetic retinopathy. OPCs also deter the deterioration of collagen, a basic building block of the skin, blood vessels, cartilage, tendons, and ligaments. The alpha-hydroxy acid in grapes helps remove superficial dead skin cells, which in turn supposedly diminishes fine wrinkles.

Of late, another compound, resveratrol, has been identified in grapes. Resvera-trol possesses significant anti-inflammatory potential and displays some ability to lower blood fats, protect the body from oxidation, and inhibit certain tumors. Grape leaves contain anywhere from 10 to 100 times more of this phytochemical than the fruit, but the seeds are possibly as rich a source as the leaves.

Dosage Options:
When OPCs were initially identified and isolated in pine bark, they were collectively known as pycnogenol. Grape seed extract may be the better source, but you'll still find pycnogenol and pine bark extracts at health food stores. 75 to 300 milligrams of grape seed extract daily for up to 3 weeks, then a daily maintenance dose of 40 to 100 milligrams.

Safety Rating: 2

Precautions:
None reported.

GREEN TEA

See "Tea" on page 210.

GUARANA *(Paullinia cupana)*

What It Is:
In Brazil, people drink brewed or carbonated guarana beverages as often as Ameri-cans drink coffee and cola—and for much the same reason: They contain a good deal of caffeine. Guarana is a perennial vine native to the Amazon region. Its dark yellow or orange red fruit contain seeds that are a bit smaller than hazelnuts. These seeds are dried, roasted, crushed, and rolled into sticks or bars, which are then con-

sumed as is or made into caffeinated drinks. Guarana initially tastes somewhat bitter and astringent, then rather sweet. It smells a little like chocolate.

Therapeutic Uses:
🍃 Arthritis, diarrhea, fatigue, headache, intestinal inflammation, migraine, nerve pain, obesity.
▦ Folk uses: Dysentery, fever, malaria, menstrual irregularities, stress.

Medicinal Properties:
Like coffee, guarana owes its therapeutic effects to caffeine, as well as to small amounts of theobromine and theophylline. (For more information on caffeine's medicinal properties, see "Coffee" on page 78.)

Dosage Options:
Five hundred to 1,000 milligrams of the dried herb or 1 to 2 grams of guarana resin or crushed seeds in a cup of hot water daily.

Safety Rating: 2

Precautions:
Guarana is generally as safe as coffee. (See the precautions under "Coffee" on page 78.)

GUGUL *(Commiphora wightii)*

What It Is:
How would the elegance of Christian literature be changed if the Bible told a tale of three wise men carrying frankincense and gugul? It might be true. The generally leafless gugul tree, native to the Middle East and India, is related to myrrh, and it, too, bleeds a gooey whitish resin, called gugul or gum guggulu. In Ayurvedic medicine, gugul is held in high regard as a treatment for arthritis and blood fat problems. And not even the most nit-picking advocate of phytochemicals can differentiate between gugul and what is supposed to be myrrh.

Therapeutic Uses:
🍃 Acne, arterial blockages, arthritis, hardening of the arteries, heart disease, high blood pressure, high cholesterol, high triglycerides, indigestion, inflammation, low libido, menstrual irregularities, obesity, sores, tissue swelling, water retention.
▦ Folk use: Gum disease.

Medicinal Properties:
Gugul's resin markedly improves your cardiovascular risk profile. According to clinical and animal studies, it not only lowers low-density lipoprotein (LDL) cholesterol and triglycerides, but it also elevates the beneficial high-density lipoprotein (HDL)

cholesterol and (at least in animals) helps reverse atherosclerotic plaque deposits. In addition, gugul deters blood clotting and protects the heart from free radical oxidative injury. It appears to accelerate the liver's processing of bad blood fats, with an assist from a little stimulation of the thyroid gland, a metabolic increase that could explain why the resin assists in weight loss. Experiments also demonstrate that the guggulsterones in this herb soothe inflammation.

Prescription Counterparts:
In India, the standardized extract, called gugulipid, is a cholesterol- and triglyceride-lowering drug that works at least as well as, and in several respects better than, such common pharmaceuticals as lovastatin (Mevacor), cholestyramine (LoCholest), and gemfibrozil (Lopid). A notable difference is that whereas the prescription medications carry a huge potential for a number of adverse reactions, including a variety of gastrointestinal disturbances, gugulipid is well-tolerated.

Dosage Options:
You want a product standardized for guggulsterones. Labels on the better supplements will indicate this potency in several different ways. Look for something that will provide 25 milligrams of guggulsterones for a dosage two or three times a day. Alternatively, 250 to 500 milligrams daily of a supplement standardized for 5 to 10 percent guggulsterones or a supplement that contains 1,200 to 1,500 milligrams of gugulipid, which should give you about 40 to 60 milligrams of guggulsterones.

Safety Rating: 2

Precautions:
All in all, rather safe. Some people might notice some belching or perhaps a skin reaction. Others might get the hiccups, a headache, or diarrhea; feel nauseous; or lose their appetite. Still others might feel restless or apprehensive. If you have diarrhea, irritable bowel syndrome, or a liver disease, be cautious about taking gugul.

GYMNEMA *(Gymnema sylvestre)*

What It Is:
A longtime treatment for diabetes in India, gymnema is a vine with egg-shaped leaves and yellow flower clusters. Indigenous to tropical Asian forests, it popped up in American health food stores only relatively recently—and for the entirely wrong reason. It was hawked as a natural "sugar blocker" that could prevent the body's absorption of the sweet stuff—thus, allegedly, preventing absorption of the calories. In truth, all gymnema can do in this regard is block your taste of sweetness (and only if applied directly to the tongue and not swallowed). The plant holds its true medicinal value for those who shouldn't be consuming sugar in the first place: It might be one of the best herbal therapies for people with diabetes.

Therapeutic Uses:

༚༚ Diabetes (types 1 and 2).

༚ High cholesterol, high triglycerides, stomachache.

▨ Folk uses: Coughing, eye inflammation, fever, obesity, scaly skin, snakebite.

Medicinal Properties:
Clinical studies and animal experiments have proved that gymnema helps control blood sugar in people who have type 1 diabetes, in which the pancreas does not secrete the sugar- and carbohydrate-metabolizing hormone insulin, or type 2 diabetes, in which the pancreas produces too little insulin or the body doesn't use the insulin efficiently. In some experiments, insulin requirements dropped by 50 percent when gymnema was used. Animal studies indicate that the plant actually regenerates insulin-secreting cells on the pancreas and stimulates insulin secretion. In a small study of 27 people with type 1 diabetes, gymnema lowered required insulin dosages, cut fasting blood sugar levels, and improved blood sugar control. In a study of 22 people with type 2 diabetes, 21 people were able to reduce their dosages of oral diabetes drugs. Five of the 21 were able to stop taking those potentially dangerous medications entirely, maintaining healthy blood sugar levels solely through the use of gymnema.

Prescription Counterparts:
People who need to give themselves insulin shots often gain weight, particularly on the parts of the body where they most frequently inject the hormone. For people with non-insulin-dependent diabetes, many standard oral drugs increase the risk of heart disease. Gymnema could drastically limit those unfortunate possibilities. One study demonstrated that it's as medicinally effective as the drug tolbutamide. Though limited, the research suggests that people with diabetes can markedly reduce their dependence on expensive, potentially dangerous pharmaceuticals.

Dosage Options:
One to 2 tablespoons of fresh leaves, 2 to 3 grams of dried leaves, 1 to 2 teaspoons of a liquid extract, or 2 to 4 grams of powdered leaves daily.

Safety Rating: 1

Precautions:
None reported. However, gymnema may increase insulin secretion in healthy, nondiabetic people—not a desirable action. If you have either type 1 or type 2 diabetes, consult an herb-savvy physician before taking gymnema and keep an even more vigilant watch on your blood sugar. Ingesting the herb very likely will demand an adjustment of insulin or other hyperglycemic medications.

HAWTHORN *(Crataegus monogyna)*

What It Is:
The tart, bright red fruit of the hawthorn looks much like a crab apple, and in certain parts of China, it's even made into candied apple–like treats. Some 200 different species of this bushy, often thorny tree grow throughout Europe and northeastern North America. From the ancient Greeks and Chinese to Native Americans and nineteenth-century folk physicians, hawthorn has been almost universally regarded as a heart tonic.

Therapeutic Uses:
🌿🌿 Cardiovascular insufficiency, hardening of the arteries, high blood pressure, irregular heart rhythm.

🌿 Acne, anemia, breathing difficulty, heart disease, high cholesterol, insomnia, palpitations, seborrhea, skin inflammation, tissue swelling, water retention.

▦ Folk uses: Buerger's disease, kidney inflammation, myocardial inflammation, rapid heart rate, slow heart rate, sore throat.

Medicinal Properties:
Although some evidence suggests that the astringent fruit might help certain skin problems, hawthorn is, for all practical purposes, mostly a cardiovascular supplement—and a supreme one at that. As clinical studies have proved, its medicinal ingredients (including proanthocyanidins and flavonoids such as quercetin, hyperoside, vitexin, vitexin-rhamnoside, and rutin) improve the heart muscle's metabolism, allowing for better contractions and a more stable rhythmic beating; dilate coronary blood vessels, permitting a larger, freer flow of blood and oxygen; deter the release of a substance called angiotensin converting enzyme (ACE), which has been identified as a cause of high blood pressure; and protect blood vessels, collagen, and other tissue from oxidizing damage.

Take the implications to heart—your heart. As a result of these pharmacologic effects, hawthorn extracts have a marked impact on angina pectoris (the chest pains caused by a dearth of blood to an overtaxed heart), atherosclerosis (the blood-blocking buildup of oxidized cholesterol inside your arteries), the artery-constricting pressure of hypertension, and the fluid buildup of congestive heart failure. Better flow of oxygen-rich blood also helps facilitate breathing.

Prescription Counterparts:
In the early stages of heart disease, hawthorn performs better than the drug digitalis and with fewer side effects. For minimal rhythmic disturbances and the initial onset of congestive heart failure, it can save the day before physicians are ready to prescribe the pharmaceutical.

Dosage Options:
Two or three 450-milligram capsules or tablets of a standardized supplement containing 100 milligrams of certified-potency hawthorn extract and a minimum of 1.8 milligrams of vitexins, 2 to 6 teaspoons of fresh hawthorn fruit, ⅛ to ¼ teaspoon of a liquid extract, or 2 teaspoons to 1 tablespoon of a leaf or fruit extract daily. Or 1 teaspoon of hawthorn tincture twice a day. You can also eat the cooked fruit or make jelly or wine with it.

Safety Rating: 3

Precautions:
Not many, although anyone with a serious heart condition should be under the care of a physician. Some people may experience a rash, nausea, some fatigue, or increased perspiration. High doses might lower blood pressure or act as a sedative. Long-term use apparently poses no problems. One stray report claimed that hawthorn might interfere with regular heart rhythm. The extract mixes well with all prescription heart medications except digitalis. Supplements may magnify the action of this drug. Although hawthorn is a food, most naturopaths do not recommend eating the fruit raw.

Hops 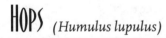 *(Humulus lupulus)*

What It Is:
Can't sleep? Fill a pillow with a bunch of hops strobili (the fruiting cones that follow the yellowish or greenish flowers) and rest your head. That cure for insomnia is almost as traditional as using hops to make beer. The plant—a close relative of stinging nettle and the *Cannabis* genus, which gives us marijuana—is native to North America, Europe, and Asia. It's always been used to soothe and settle. Some thought it worked too well. In fifteenth- and sixteenth-century England, it was banned for inducing not only sedation but also sadness. Only in the seventeenth century did hops become a common ingredient in English beer.

Therapeutic Uses:
ᕦᕤ Anxiety, insomnia, nervousness, restlessness.
ᕤ Cramps, diarrhea, indigestion, infections, lack of appetite, neuroses, nerve pain, stress, tuberculosis.

✴ Folk uses: Arthritis, boils, bruises, colitis, coughing, depression, leprosy, menstrual irregularities, priapism.

Medicinal Properties:
A number of phytochemicals in hops possess sedative and muscle-relaxing qualities. Other compounds depress the central nervous system. The bitterness helps trigger appetite.

Dosage Options:
One 500-milligram capsule or tablet, ⅛ to ½ teaspoon of a liquid extract, or 2 to 6 teaspoons of fresh flowers daily. Or try ¼ to ½ teaspoon of hops tincture up to three times a day.

Safety Rating: 3

Precautions:
Some sensitive people might experience a mild skin or respiratory allergy from direct contact with hops or from inhalation of hops pollen. If you've been diagnosed with depression, think twice about taking the herb because of its sedative action.

HOREHOUND, WHITE *(Marrubium vulgare)*

See "White Horehound" on page 220.

HORSE CHESTNUT *(Aesculus hippocastanum)*

What It Is:
Indigenous to Albania, Bulgaria, and other Balkan countries, the horse chestnut tree and its nuts (seeds, actually) supposedly soothe equine respiratory afflictions—hence the common name that has carried over to some of the other dozen varieties, including the one we know as the buckeye. The research is inconclusive as to whether the other members of the family offer as much therapeutic potential as true European horse chestnut. The tree can grow up to 100 feet tall. It sports a number of white flowers dotted with flecks of red or yellow and thorny seedpods that split open in the fall to yield their nuts. Although the bark, leaves, and flowers have been used in folk remedies, the nuts' pulp contains the strongest concentration of medicinal ingredients. Don't roast these chestnuts on an open fire during the next holiday season; they're unrelated to the oak family's sweet chestnut. The bitter-tasting horse chestnut, plucked right from the tree, is not edible; some say it's poisonous. Processed horse chestnut, though, has been consumed as a food.

Therapeutic Uses:

༈༈ Chronic venous insufficiency, hemorrhoids, sunburn, swelling, varicose veins.

༈ Anal inflammation, arthritis, blood clots, bruises, carpal tunnel syndrome, cellulite, disc inflammation, dizziness, flu, headache, hematoma, itching, leg cramps, malaria, menstrual pain, muscular paralysis (palsy), pimples, prostatitis, sores, thrombophlebitis, tissue swelling, water retention, wounds, wrinkles.

▦ Folk uses: Asthma, backache, colds, congestion, coughing, diarrhea, dysentery, eczema, fever, indigestion, intestinal disease, liver disease, lupus, nerve pain, phlebitis, sprains, stomach disease and inflammation.

Medicinal Properties:

Horse chestnut's value is vascular. It bucks up weak, leaky veins and capillaries that allow blood to ooze out, pool under the skin, and give rise to problems such as hemorrhoids, varicose veins, spider veins, and other circulatory disorders indicative of a lack of sufficient blood flow. It also counteracts related inflammation and cell-destroying oxidation. The antioxidant, capillary-toughening action also might help fend off two aesthetic irritants—cellulite and wrinkles. Scientists have identified one phytochemical, aescin, as the key to horse chestnut's therapeutic secrets. Although aescin is an active ingredient, it is certainly not the only one. Whole-herb extracts possess more anti-inflammatory punch than aescin alone, thanks to other compounds as rutin.

Dosage Options:

One 257-milligram standardized supplement providing 18 to 22 percent aescin twice a day (or, calculated another way, enough to provide about 100 milligrams of aescin). Other dosage options include ½ to 1¼ teaspoons of a standardized liquid bark or fruit extract or 1 to 3 teaspoons of horse chestnut tincture daily. Do not ingest any preparation made from horse chestnut seeds unless it was prescribed by an herb-savvy physician. The seeds are poisonous unless processed properly (see "Precautions").

Safety Rating: 2

Precautions:

Except for the seeds, few side effects have been reported. The aesculin in horse chestnut could cause a skin reaction upon contact. Pure aescin can be toxic to the kidneys and cause intestinal upset or vomiting, impaired liver function, spasms, or even shock. Intravenous preparations have caused rare cases of kidney or liver poisoning. Consuming too many seeds (perhaps as few as five for a child) can cause diarrhea, flushing, mental or visual disturbances, severe thirst, vomiting, and, at the most extreme, death.

HORSERADISH (Armoracia rusticana)

What It Is:
Horseradish is pungently persistent in more ways than taste. Cut off the top of the plant, including the top of its roots, and a new top (and new roots) will grow. Although the weed doesn't reseed itself, it nevertheless reappears season after season. If you ever plant horseradish and then change your mind, you'll have to get rid of every trace of the roots, or the plant, with its large (a foot or two long), tongue-shaped, similarly pungent leaves, will grow anew. In early times, horseradish was well-known and often eaten among the Germans and Dutch, but it wasn't accepted as a common condiment in England until the sixteenth century or so. The name has no equine implications. In early England, *horse* also meant "coarse," as in inedible.

Therapeutic Uses:
🌱🌱 Bronchitis, coughing, mucous membrane inflammation, muscle pain, respiratory disease, urinary tract infections.
🌱 Arthritis, colds, congestion, cystitis, rhinitis, sinus infections, stones, urinary pain.
▦ Folk uses: Allergies, colic, dental plaque, flu, gallbladder inflammation, gout, indigestion, lack of appetite, liver disease, sciatica, sore throat, tissue swelling, water retention, worms, wounds.

Medicinal Properties:
Most of horseradish's therapeutic properties come from pungent sulfur-containing compounds called isothiocyanates, as well as another phytochemical called sulforaphane. Both kill germs and stimulate blood flow (especially to the skin), but they pack a wallop when it comes to opening up the sinuses and blowing out congestion.

Dosage Options:
One to 2 tablespoons of fresh roots daily, ½ teaspoon or so of horseradish tincture three times a day, or as much horseradish dressing as your tastebuds and sinuses can stand. You also can make a horseradish plaster and apply it topically. I have enjoyed horseradish sauce sandwiches as sinus openers.

Safety Rating: 2

Precautions:
In reasonable amounts, none reported. People with gastritis, kidney disease, or ulcers should avoid horseradish because of its irritant action. Don't feed it to children younger than 4. Some people might be allergic to the herb's glucosinolates.

HORSETAIL (*Equisetum arvense*)

What It Is:
Is that green scouring pad on your kitchen sink worn-out? If so, go out and pick some horsetail. This plant, a flowerless leftover from prehistoric times, is rich in silica, a natural abrasive. Smart campers across North America still pick wild horsetail to scour dirty pots and pans after they've cooked dinner over the fire. (No wonder it's also called scouring rush.) Once the maturing plant forms and releases cases of reproductive spores, it grows bushy stems that resemble a horse's tail.

Therapeutic Uses:
🌿🌿 Bladder stones, burns, cystitis, gravel, inflammation, kidney stones, respiratory problems, tissue swelling, urinary tract infections, urinary inflammation, water retention, wounds.

🌿 Brittle nails, infections, kidney disease, prostatitis, stomach disease, nosebleeds, uterine hemorrhage.

▨ Folk uses: Arthritis, bed-wetting, bloody urine, constipation, eye inflammation, fractures, frostbite, gallbladder problems, gonorrhea, gout, hair loss and other problems, hemorrhoids, incontinence, osteoporosis, sprains, stomach disease, swelling, tuberculosis.

Medicinal Properties:
Aside from scraping gunk from kitchen utensils, silicon (and, by extension, horsetail) is an underappreciated, health-promoting mineral. Advocates point out that silicon contributes to healthy bones, cartilage, tendons, and connective tissue. We apparently need it, and it disappears from our bodies as we get older. Some French researchers assert that silicon could assist in preventing osteoporosis and in speeding the healing of bone fractures.

Dosage Options:
Three 350-milligram capsules three times a day, one 500-milligram standardized supplement twice a day, or ½ to 1 teaspoon of a liquid extract or tincture daily. Or make a daily tea by steeping 1 to 4 grams of the dried herb in a cup of hot water. Add about a teaspoon of sugar, bring to a boil, and let simmer for up to 3 hours. The sugar will extract more of horsetail's active ingredients. Strain the tea before you drink it.

Safety Rating: 1

Precautions:
Not many, if any, with rational use. Don't give horsetail to children. Some kids who have ingested horsetail end up with a condition that resembles nicotine poisoning. (Some horsetail species do contain nicotine.) Don't take it if you have heart disease or kidney disease.

HYDRANGEA *(Hydrangea arborescens)*

What It Is:
Found in marshy areas along the East Coast of the United States, hydrangea features small white flowers and a rough bark that peels off easily—hence one of the plant's other names, seven barks. Native Americans and early settlers used hydrangea's roots to treat gravel, stones in the urinary tract, and other calcified accumulations in the body.

Therapeutic Uses:
🐾 Allergies, inflammation, tumors.
▦ Folk uses: Bladder stones, bronchitis, burns, cancer, cystitis, gallbladder problems, gravel, indigestion, infections, kidney inflammation, kidney stones, muscle pain, prostatitis, sprains, stones, urethritis, urinary stones.

Medicinal Properties:
Little hard science exists to validate the folk uses of hydrangea. It does contain quercetin, rutin, and other flavonoids that, among other actions, help reduce inflammation and lower the risk of tumor growth. Synthetic derivatives of one active ingredient, hydrangenol, may fight allergies and act as an antihistamine.

Dosage Options:
One-half to 1 teaspoon of a liquid root extract up to three times a day, 1 tablespoon of fresh roots daily, or ½ to 2 teaspoons of a root tincture daily.

Safety Rating: 1

Precautions:
Don't take hydrangea for too long, and don't take too much. It contains cyanogen-like compounds. Large doses could cause dizziness and a tight feeling in the chest. The plant's hydrangin might cause intestinal or stomach inflammation in some people.

HYSSOP *(Hyssopus officinalis)*

What It Is:
Because of its strong fragrance, hyssop has been used in everything from colognes to liqueurs. Also used since the days of ancient Greece to ease bronchitis and other respiratory inflammation, it's found in various cold nostrums. The plant's tall, erect stems are topped by clusters of little, bluish purple flowers. Indigenous to Europe and Asia, this member of the mint family now grows naturally across much of North America.

Therapeutic Uses:

🌿🌿 Colds, fever, gallbladder problems, herpes, liver disease.

🌿 Bronchitis, chronic venous insufficiency, cold sores, coughing, gas, hemorrhoids, HIV, inflammation, sore throat, tissue swelling, varicose veins, water retention.

▨ Folk uses: Arthritis, asthma, colic, eye inflammation, frostbite prevention, gout, heart disease, hoarseness, indigestion, intestinal inflammation, lung disease, menstrual pain, mucous membrane inflammation, obesity, wounds.

Medicinal Properties:

The plant's essential oils apparently help break up phlegm and soothe irritated mucous membranes in the respiratory tract. The phytochemical marrubiin also helps break up congestion. Two other chemical constituents, diosmin and ursolic acid, relieve inflammation. Hyssop is our best source of diosmin, which also protects the capillaries and eases tissue swelling and water retention. In laboratory experiments, hyssop extracts have shown much promise in inhibiting both the herpes virus and HIV, the virus that causes AIDS.

Dosage Options:

One to 2 teaspoons of the dried herb in a cup of hot water up to three times a day or ½ to 1 teaspoon of a liquid extract daily.

Safety Rating: 3

Precautions:

For the whole herb and herb extracts, none reported. Hyssop's volatile oils, like all volatile oils, are toxic, capable of causing spasms and convulsions.

IPECAC *(Cephaelis ipecacuanha)*

What It Is:
In Colombia and elsewhere in Central and South America, people chew the roots to repel insects and treat amoeba infections. Don't do this at home. Save the syrup of this low-lying, shade-loving, berry-bearing tropical evergreen for the only reason it should be in your medicine cabinet: as a vomit-inducing emergency treatment for poisoning until you can get to the hospital. The name comes from the plant's Portuguese moniker, *ipecacuanha* from the native term *i-pe-kaa-guéne,* said to translate as "roadside sick-making plant."

Therapeutic Uses:
🌿🌿 Croup, poisoning.
🌿 Amoeba infections, bronchitis, coughing, diarrhea, dysentery, whooping cough.
▦ Folk uses: Flu, morning sickness.

Medicinal Properties:
Ironically, very small doses of ipecac inhibit vomiting and may even curb morning sickness.

Dosage Options:
As little as ¼ teaspoon of ipecac syrup, a root tincture, or a liquid root extract will make you throw up. So will 1 to 2 grams of dried root or 25 to 100 milligrams of powdered ipecac.

Safety Rating: 1

Precautions:
Ipecac is a one-time, first-aid herb. Extremely large dosages can provoke convulsions, erode the mucous membranes lining the gastrointestinal tract, lower blood pressure, raise heart rate, cause respiratory problems, and induce shock or even coma.

JUNIPER *(Juniperus communis)*

What It Is:
If you've ever had a shot of gin, you've had a little juniper juice. The bluish black berries are the liquor's main flavoring ingredient. The berries technically are cones, which befit a shrub that, with its pointy, needlelike leaves, sort of resembles a pine tree. It's indigenous to North America and Europe.

Therapeutic Uses:
🍂🍂 Lack of appetite, stones, urinary tract infections.
🍂 Arthritis, bladder disease and inflammation, diabetes, flu, gas, gout, heartburn, heart disease, herpes, high blood pressure, indigestion, infections, prostate enlargement (benign).
▦ Folk uses: Aches, belching, bronchitis, cancer, colds, colic, congestion, coughing, cramps, intestinal inflammation, menstrual pain, muscle pain, nerve pain, neuroses, psoriasis, sores, snakebite, stomachache, worms.

Medicinal Properties:
Juniper is a good diuretic and urinary antiseptic, helpful against urinary tract infections. It also contains a powerful virus-killing substance, deoxypodophyllotoxin, and other phytochemicals that can fight herpes and influenza.

Prescription Counterparts:
In tests involving lab rats, juniper berry extract displayed more anti-inflammatory strength than indomethacin. A tumor-fighting substance in juniper called podophyllotoxin is potent against malaria, too.

Dosage Options:
One teaspoon of juniper syrup daily, ½ to 1 teaspoon of a liquid fruit extract three times a day, ¼ to ½ teaspoon of a fruit tincture three times a day, 1 teaspoon of fresh fruit daily, or 1 teaspoon of juniper berries in 1 cup of hot water three or four times a day for up to 4 weeks.

Safety Rating: 1

Precautions:
Don't take juniper for more than 4 to 6 weeks, and don't take it if you have a kidney problem. Excessive dosages or prolonged use might lead to kidney damage. Topical use of juniper's essential oil can inflame or burn the skin.

K

Kava-Kava *(Piper methysticum)*

What It Is:

In America, people like to wind down, fight stress, and generally take the edge off with cocktails, sleeping pills, and antidepressants. In Polynesia and the Pacific Ocean islands, where kava-kava (or just kava) is indigenous, they calm down with this pepper-family member. You can chew a few of the shrub's leaves to relax, but the best antistress medicine is in the roots, which are most often dried, ground, and used to make a tea. It's a perfect antithesis (and antidote) to coffee—and about as safe, too.

Therapeutic Uses:

❧❧ Anxiety, insomnia, nervousness, restlessness, stress.

❧ Cramps, dizziness, earache, epilepsy, fatigue, headache, hyperactivity, indigestion, menopause, menstrual pain, migraine, muscle pain, palpitations, stomachache, toothache.

▣ Folk uses: Arthritis, bed-wetting, bronchitis, colds, colic, coughing, debility, eye inflammation, gallbladder problems, gonorrhea, gout, hemorrhoids, incontinence, kidney inflammation, lack of appetite, leprosy, mucous membrane inflammation, nerve pain, skin problems, sore throat, urinary tract infections, vaginitis, venereal disease, water retention.

Medicinal Properties:

Phytochemicals called kavalactones provide kava's gentle stress-beating, muscle-relaxing influence. Each produces a somewhat different physiologic effect in the body, and all of them working together are better than any one of them acting alone. Kava also possesses a curious affinity for the genitourinary tract, especially in women; it relaxes the uterus, making it notably helpful against menstrual cramps. And because chewing on a couple of kava leaves numbs your mouth, it might alleviate toothaches and other oral afflictions.

Prescription Counterparts:

Several comparative studies have proved solidly that kava extracts reduce stress and anxiety at least as well as popular prescription tranquilizers such as diazepam (Valium) and other benzodiazepines. The herb also doesn't impair mental reaction, upset the stomach, or present the same strong potential for addiction as those drugs. In one study, mental function actually improved. Other research has shown that two of the kavalactones together provide as much analgesic relief as 200 milligrams of aspirin, with no risk of irritating the stomach.

Dosage Options:
Most people will probably want to take kava at the end of the day or an hour or so before bedtime, just to relax or to help them fall asleep. More nervous, stressed-out, or anxious people might want to take it several times a day. Possible dosages include 1 teaspoon of powdered root in a tea up to three times a day, a standardized supplement containing 250 milligrams of certified-potency kava extract providing 75 milligrams of kavalactones either three times a day or 1 hour before bedtime, or ½ to 1 teaspoon of a liquid root extract one or more times a day or 1 hour before bedtime.

Safety Rating: 2

Precautions:
Very few side effects with reasonable use. Kava is not, as some people have claimed, a narcotic or a hallucinogen, nor is it addictive. A few sensitive people might experience some dizziness, a headache, or a stomachache. Others might notice a lower libido while under kava's mellowing influence. Continuous overuse or chronic abuse could tint your skin yellow, a harmless, reversible condition called kawism or kava dermatitis. Continuous abuse of inordinately high dosages could cause a more serious dermatologic reaction—scaly eruptions on the skin known as kani or kava dermopathy. The mouth-numbing sensation produced by chewing the leaves or roots also is harmless and temporary. Kava can magnify the effects of alcohol, tranquilizers, barbiturates, and central nervous system depressants. Looked at another way, kava may be able to help you lessen your need for such medications. Talk to your doctor about possibly using kava to reduce your drug dosages.

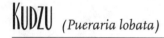

KUDZU *(Pueraria lobata)*

What It Is:
Plant some kudzu, and it'll spread like crazy. You'll find kudzu across millions of acres in the southeastern United States, where it was introduced to control erosion. It's native to Asia, however, where it has thrived for more than a thousand years. Kudzu root, which can grow as big as an average-size male, once served as a primary source of starch in China and Japan until the introduction of sweet potatoes. It also used to be a traditional treatment for diarrhea and dysentery. Today the starch is commonly used as a thickener in commercially processed foods. Kudzu might be missing a higher calling, though, for science has found a few intriguing medicinal possibilities.

Therapeutic Uses:

🌿 Alcoholism, breast cancer, chest pain, cirrhosis and other liver diseases, deafness, high blood pressure, irregular heart rhythm, leukemia, osteoporosis.

▓ Folk uses: Allergies, breast inflammation, colds, diabetes, diarrhea, dysentery, flu, gastritis, hangover, headache, hives, intestinal inflammation, measles, psoriasis, sores, sore throat, swelling.

Medicinal Properties:

An animal experiment conducted in the early 1990s asserted that extracts of kudzu root's isoflavones, particularly daidzein and daidzin, can curb the urge to consume alcohol. Other research has concluded that extracts may strengthen the liver's ability to fend off damage from toxins and even help the organ regenerate itself. The isoflavone genistein reportedly fights leukemia and deters tumor development and growth. Kudzu root is apparently richer in these estrogenic phytochemicals than soybean. Flavonoid-like constituents improve blood flow through coronary arteries, as well as veins and capillaries. As a result, kudzu extracts are used to treat angina pectoris chest pains and high blood pressure, including such hypertensive symptoms as dizziness, headache, and ringing in the ears.

Prescription Counterparts:

More research needs to be done to determine kudzu's ability to treat alcoholism, but it might be worth considering before resorting to mainstream medicine's pharmaceutical alternatives, disulfiram (Antabuse) and naltrexone hydrochloride (ReVia). Antabuse inflicts a violent physical reaction (headache, vomiting, chest pain, difficulty breathing, and blurred vision, to name a few) upon ingesting any quantity of alcohol, even if it's in food, over-the-counter medicines, or an aftershave. ReVia is targeted more to heroin and other opioid addictions, but some research shows that it also helps deter the desire to drink and lowers relapse rates if used as part of a more comprehensive antialcohol therapy. Like alcoholism, both drugs can cause or magnify liver problems.

Ipriflavone, a relatively new synthetic supplement derived from soy isoflavones and marketed as good for building bone density, is converted in the body in part to daidzein. Ipriflavone may temporarily elevate liver enzymes and affect the body's ability to metabolize some medications. Kudzu might be a safer alternative.

Dosage Options:

Enough of a standardized kudzu root extract to provide 3 milligrams of daidzin per day. Follow the recommendations on the supplement label.

Safety Rating: 2

Precautions:

None reported.

LAVENDER (*Lavandula*, various species)

What It Is:
The pleasantly powerful, distinctive fragrance of this pretty, purple-flowered plant has been popular since the earliest days of recorded history. The ancient Romans scented their baths with lavender, almost certainly giving rise to the plant's name: The Latin verb *lavare* means "to wash." The ancient Egyptians also used lavender as a perfume. Good ingredients never go out of style. You'll still find lavender oil in soaps, perfumes, and sachets.

Therapeutic Uses:
🌿🌿 Gas, insomnia, intestinal disease, lack of appetite, nervousness, restlessness, stomachache, stomach disease.
🌿 Diabetes, gallbladder problems, gas, indigestion, labor, wounds.
▦ Folk uses: Cancer, colds, dementia, depression, headache, menstrual pain, psoriasis, skin problems, stress.

Medicinal Properties:
Lavender's soothing, sedating phytochemicals readily absorb into the skin, including the sensitive membranes inside the nose. That's why even the scent of lavender oil tends to calm and relax. Chemicals in the oil, including linalool and linalyl alcohol, appear to slow nerve impulses, reducing irritability and excitement and helping to deaden pain.

Dosage Options:
One to 2 teaspoons of dried lavender flowers in a cup of hot water several times a day and particularly at night, ½ to 1 teaspoon of lavender tincture daily, or 1 ounce or more of dried lavender flowers sprinkled in your bathwater. Alternatively, you can put a couple of drops of lavender oil in your bath or rub a drop or two on your skin. Do not ingest the oil.

Safety Rating: 2

Precautions:
None reported, but don't ingest lavender oil.

LEMON BALM (Melissa officinalis)

What It Is:
The genus name, *Melissa*, comes from the Greek word meaning "bee." Long ago, beekeepers rubbed its scented, serrated leaves on hives to attract the little stingers. A member of the mint family, the herb is native to the Mediterranean and certain areas of Asia but now exudes its distinct lemony aroma over much of the eastern and central United States.

Therapeutic Uses:
ᕊᕊ Cold sores, gas, gastric spasms, indigestion, insomnia, intestinal disease, nervousness, stomach disease.

ᕊ Alzheimer's disease, colds, headache, herpes, mumps, muscle tone problems, nerve pain, palpitations, restlessness, shingles, hyperthyroidism (Graves' disease), tumors.

▦ Folk uses: Anxiety, bronchitis, bug bites, heart disease, high blood pressure, hysteria, melancholy, menstrual pain, migraine, mucous membrane inflammation, nausea, wounds.

Medicinal Properties:
The tannins and other polyphenols in lemon balm extracts deter certain viruses, notably those that cause mumps and herpes. These phytochemicals apparently nudge out the virus for spots on cellular receptors that the viruses seem to favor. That little game of medicinal musical chairs strands the bugs, rendering them unable to infect the body and spread. Lemon balm extract, at least when administered intravenously, also helps normalize thyroid function, particularly against a hyperactive condition called Graves' disease. The phytochemicals block antibodies of the disease from latching onto the thyroid gland. The herb decreases both blood and pituitary levels of thyroid-stimulating hormone, thus lowering the gland's output. Finally, the terpenes in lemon balm tend to relax you and help you fall asleep.

Prescription Counterparts:
One study demonstrated that a cream containing about 700 milligrams of lemon balm sped the healing of herpes sores by several days, comparable in effect to the pharmaceutical acyclovir (Zovirax). This common prescription drug can cause or contribute to kidney impairment, and its other side effects include nausea, vomiting, a sense of malaise, and disruptions in the menstrual cycle.

Dosage Options:
One-half to 1 teaspoon of a liquid extract daily, ½ to 1 ½ teaspoons of lemon balm tincture three times a day, or 1 to 3 teaspoons of the dried herb in a cup of hot water at least once a day. For cold sores, if you can't find a lemon balm cream, apply the tea directly to the sore as often as you'd like. The used tea leaves also can be applied to the lesion.

Safety Rating: 3

Precautions:

None reported. Some herbalists claim that lemon balm's essential oils could raise ocular pressure, a concern of anyone with or at risk for glaucoma. Other experts dispute the plant's value in treating Graves' disease, some even saying that it will exacerbate the condition.

LICORICE *(Glycyrrhiza glabra)*

What It Is:

Licorice was used therapeutically in ancient China and Rome, mostly for respiratory complaints and intestinal woes. Ever since, the plant's roots have been used for these conditions and more, with an ever-growing mountain of scientific evidence to back up the applications. Some 20 different licorice species grow in parts of Europe, Asia, North America, South America, and Australia. The plant typically sports small, pointy leaves and flower clusters. Licorice derives its common name from *liquirtia*, a Latin term based on the plant's original Greek name, *glukos riza*, or "sweet root." The active ingredient, glycyrrhizin, is 50 times sweeter than sugar, but it has an aftertaste that puts a lot of people off. Perhaps that's one reason why, at least in the United States, those "ropes" of licorice candy usually contain more anise than licorice.

Therapeutic Uses:

🍂🍂 Bronchitis, coughing, mucous membrane inflammation, respiratory disease, stomach inflammation, ulcers.

🍂 Addison's disease, arthritis, asthma, cataracts, caries, central nervous system disease, chronic fatigue syndrome, colds, congestion, diabetes, encephalitis, flu, gallbladder problems, hepatitis, herpes, HIV, indigestion, kidney disease, lichen planus, lupus, malaria, overeating, polycystic ovary syndrome, prostate enlargement (benign), retinopathy, sore throat, thrush, tuberculosis, urinary tract infections, vaginitis, yeast infections.

▨ Folk uses: Appendicitis, boils, canker sores, colic, constipation, consumption, cramps, depression, diphtheria, dizziness, earache, eczema, epilepsy, eye inflammation, fibromyalgia, heartburn, heart disease, hemorrhoids, kidney stones, lack of appetite, menstrual pain, oral inflammation, snakebite, tetanus, viral hepatitis.

Medicinal Properties for Licorice:

Licorice's phytochemical components are among the best studied (and most complicated) in all of herbal medicine. Two major ingredients are glycyrrhizin and glycyrrhetinic acid, but even without them, the herb, in the form of deglycyrrhizinated licorice (DGL), retains the healing powers of licoricone and related flavonoids, triterpenoids, lignans, and other phytochemicals. Let's look at each.

Medicinal Properties for Whole Licorice Root Extract:

Inflammation. Glycyrrhizin blocks prostaglandin production and inflammation. Although it supports the body's release of cortisol, it also inhibits some of the more detrimental side effects of that natural hormone's presence, such as increasing cholesterol synthesis in the liver and blocking the work of the adrenal glands and thymus. Topically, it's a very good treatment for tendinitis, bursitis, gum inflammation, and such autoimmune inflammatory reactions as psoriasis.

Viral and bacterial infections. Some 30 percent of licorice's dry weight consists of antibacterial substances, and its saponins improve the body's ability to use other antibacterial compounds. Licorice also soothes irritated mucous membranes and contains nine different natural expectorants to break up phlegm and ease coughing. This alone makes it effective against colds and the flu. But there's more: Good scientific evidence illustrates that licorice fights viruses, including Epstein-Barr, herpes, hepatitis, and HIV. Glycyrrhizin prods the immune system into secreting more interferon, a basic antiviral chemical that prevents infectious foes from taking hold inside the body. It inhibits the villainous viral invasion in which the bug penetrates a cell and changes its genetic makeup to replicate and spread.

In the liver, licorice extract protects the organ from viral hepatitis. In the mouth, it heals canker sores, with significant improvement in just a day for 75 percent of one study's participants and complete healing 2 days later. And it fights HIV, as illustrated by an experiment involving people with hemophilia who apparently contracted HIV from blood transfusions; a month's worth of glycyrrhizin supplements markedly reduced concentrations of the virus in their blood. During the course of the 7-year experiment, none of the eight licorice users got AIDS; two people in the comparison group did.

Sex hormones. Licorice offers something for both men and women. For men, it helps inhibit the conversion of testosterone into dihydrotestosterone, a form of the male hormone implicated in hair loss and prostate enlargement. For women, it appears either to raise or reduce estrogen levels, depending on the body's need.

Sugar metabolism. Licorice's isoliquiritigenin, glycyrrhizin, and glycyrrhetinic acid help prevent the buildup (especially in the eye's lens, the spine's sciatic nerve, and the bloodstream) of a form of sugar called sorbitol, which figures in many of the complications of diabetes, including cataracts and vision deterioration, nerve damage, and kidney malfunction. In this regard, isoliquiritigenin works like pharmaceuticals known as aldose reductase inhibitors, which are prescribed for these conditions.

Medicinal Properties for Deglycyrrhizinated Licorice:

Licorice occasionally thrusts a two-edged sword into your herbal medicine cabinet. The large doses sometimes necessary to generate a therapeutic effect can cause side effects, including high blood pressure, water retention, tissue swelling, weight gain, headache, lethargy, and skewed potassium and sodium levels. The side effects result from increasing levels of cortisol and other adrenal hormones. There is one instance in which the side effects are a welcome blessing: Addison's disease, in which the adrenal glands don't secrete enough cortisol and aldosterone, leaving you weak and emaciated, among other consequences.

Because of the adverse reactions, those who like to tinker with nature decided to strip licorice of its glycyrrhizin and glycyrrhetinic acid and see what healing power remained from the licoricone and related flavonoids, triterpenoids, lignans, and other phytochemicals. The effort has proved successful in treating ulcers and related stomach problems. The first drug demonstrated to encourage the healing of peptic ulcers was derived from whole licorice. DGL works just as well, advocates of the altered preparation claim. They say that besides quelling spasms and reducing stomach acid (take heed, heartburn sufferers), DGL protects and promotes the cells that line the intestinal tract, boosting blood flow to them and lengthening their lives. It also spares the stomach from aspirin's erosive effect. Despite the positive reports, some phytomedicinal experts and other herbal purists are uncomfortable with DGL and remain skeptical of its worth, believing that this version doesn't completely lose its potential for side effects but does lose many of its medicinal attributes.

Prescription Counterparts:

According to comparative studies, DGL works just as well for ulcers as the popular prescription antacids cimetidine (Tagamet) and ranitidine hydrochloride (Zantac). Yet the herb carries none of the risks of the synthetic drugs. By reducing gastric secretions, those drugs disturb normal digestion. In so doing, they also change the makeup and function of the cells lining the gastrointestinal tract. That partly explains why fans of the pharmaceuticals, which don't have this effect, suffer ulcer relapses or undergo operations more frequently than do users of DGL.

For curbing a cough, oral doses of glycyrrhetinic acid are just as good as codeine, according to research. As for psoriasis and other inflammatory problems (such as bursitis and tendinitis), licorice extracts are just as effective as hydrocortisone creams. Herbal preparations won't cause weight gain, indigestion, or insomnia, as hydrocortisone can. Nor will they render you more vulnerable to infections, another endearing trait of hydrocortisone. What's more, if you wish to use the pharmaceutical, you will get better results if you take it along with some licorice.

Dosage Options:

One to three capsules standardized to provide 200 milligrams of certified-potency licorice root extract and 50 milligrams of glycyrrhizinic acid daily. Other daily options include 200 to 600 milligrams of glycyrrhizin, ½ to 1 teaspoon of a liquid extract, 2 to 4 tablespoons of fresh roots, or ½ to 1 teaspoon of licorice tincture three times a day. For ulcers, 380 milligrams of DGL three times a day.

Safety Rating: 2

Precautions:

Licorice has gotten a bad rap from many medical authorities, mostly Americans. This herb possesses significant medicinal potential and should be regarded with the same cautious optimism as any other medicinal agent: good if used wisely, bad if used inappropriately. With moderate use in reasonable amounts, most people need not fear licorice. Stick with supplements of the whole herb, not isolated extracts of this or that glycyrrhizin component. For an ulcer, use DGL; you'll avoid side effects even if you take big dosages.

For therapeutic applications that require glycyrrhizin, some herbal experts say that you shouldn't take it longer than a month or so without seeing a doctor. Taking more than 50 grams of licorice root a day can elevate blood pressure, lower potassium levels, and cause water retention, among other problems. Given these potential problems, you probably shouldn't take the herb if you have hypertension, kidney problems, liver problems, diabetes, or heart disease.

LINDEN *(Tilia, various species)*

What It Is:
Many of the floral decorations in England's St. Paul Cathedral and Windsor Castle were carved from a species of this tree's wood, which is light and allows intricately cut detail. The medicine, though, is in the yellowish white flowers, which are highly fragrant and yield a great-tasting honey. A number of *Tilia* species exist, each with somewhat different herbal properties and all difficult to tell apart. Some call the tree linden; others call it lime; still others, mostly Americans, call it basswood.

Therapeutic Uses:
🍃🍃 Bronchitis, colds, coughing.
🍃 Anxiety, chills, earache, flu, infections, sore throat.
▨ Folk uses: Cellulitis (a deep, spreading tissue inflammation), convulsions, diarrhea, fever, gallbladder problems, hardening of the arteries, headache, high blood pressure, hysteria, indigestion, intestinal disease, migraine, mucous membrane inflammation, nervousness, premenstrual tension.

Medicinal Properties:
Linden's phytochemicals quell spasms, encourage urination, and may be somewhat sedating. They're also good for inducing perspiration, as when you have a cold or the flu and need to break a fever.

Dosage Options:
One-half to 1 teaspoon of a liquid flower extract, ¼ to ½ teaspoon of a flower tincture, or 1 to 2 teaspoons of dried linden flowers in a cup of hot water daily.

Safety Rating: 2

Precautions:
None reported with normal use. Excessive use could damage the heart.

LOBELIA *(Lobelia inflata)*

What It Is:
Native Americans used to smoke the jagged-edged leaves of this native American plant, which grows across much of the continental United States. They did so to ease asthma, giving it the name asthma weed. More recently, people looking for cheap, legal highs have smoked this weed, which is also known as Indian tobacco, or have drunk lobelia tea. It reportedly stimulates and relaxes simultaneously, while also instilling a sense of mental clarity. Lobelia, whose yellowish green leaves taste as bitter as tobacco when chewed, has been used to relieve nicotine withdrawal symptoms. Another quality of the plant is evident from two of its other names: pukeweed and vomitwort.

Therapeutic Uses:
🐾 Alzheimer's disease, asthma, bronchitis, coughing, laryngitis, nicotine addiction, sore throat, whooping cough.

▩ Folk uses: Arthritis, boils, bruises, bug bites, colds, fever, heart disease, muscle pain and inflammation, poison ivy, ringworm, sores, sprains.

Medicinal Properties:
The lobeline in lobelia acts much like nicotine, although it's less potent. It stimulates the central nervous system and speeds respiration. It also helps break up mucus and facilitates coughing.

Dosage Options:
Five to 15 drops tincture four times a day, 100 milligrams of the leaf.

Safety Rating: 1

Precautions:
Lobelia contains several hazardous compounds and has been known to cause death. As little as ½ to 1 gram of the leaves can be toxic; 4 grams can be fatal. Side effects resemble those of nicotine and can include nausea, vomiting, diarrhea, and dizziness. An overdose can lead to depression, profuse cold sweats, stupor, tremors, convulsions, coma, and death.

M

MA HUANG *(Ephedra, various species)*

See "Ephedra" on page 94.

MALABAR TAMARIND *(Garcinia cambogia)*

What It Is:
In botany, malamar tamarind is a small, round-crowned, darkly and densely leaved tree that produces tart, highly acidic, yellow fruits that often turn red. In the supplement industry, it's hugely hyped as a weight loss aid, promoted far and beyond any proven therapeutic ability. The hydroxycitric acid (HCA) in the fruit (also known as brindle berry and garcinia) supposedly curbs appetite, speeds the burning of fat, and slows adipose accumulation around the waist. Studies have cast doubt on these claims. The fruit is held in no such special regard in its native India, where it's commonly found in the nation's western forests. People include the dried rind in chutney and curry dishes. It's also quite good for preserving fish, polishing gold and silver, and helping rubber to coagulate.

Therapeutic Uses:
🍃 High cholesterol, high triglycerides, obesity.
▦ Folk uses: Arthritis, indigestion, oral disease.

Medicinal Properties:
The research on HCA's ability to win the battle of the bulge has been, at best, mixed. In lab rats, HCA has curbed appetite, reduced triglycerides, and lowered body weight. In test tube experiments, it has reduced or inhibited the synthesis of cholesterol. In studies involving people, the jury is still out.

Prescription Counterparts:
The pharmaceutical fen-phen (a name for the combination of two weight loss drugs shown to have significant health consequences for users) enjoyed only a short reign, yanked off pharmacy shelves because of its health risks. HCA is undoubtedly safer, but its efficacy remains suspect.

Dosage Options:
Supplements (all of which are patented formulations) typically call for taking 1,500 milligrams of extracted HCA in divided doses over the course of the day, sometimes along with chromium picolinate, the amino acid L-carnitine, or caffeine.

Safety Rating: 2

Precautions:
None reported.

MARSHMALLOW *(Althaea officinalis)*

What It Is:
No, the plant doesn't grow puffy white blobs of creamy goo that are good for toasting. Nor does it sprout little yellow "peeps" around Easter. There's no actual marshmallow in commercially sold marshmallow treats. Real marshmallow, native to Europe and also found in various parts of the United States, is so named because it's a member of the mallow family and tends to favor a marshy habitat. It is a tall herb with short serrated leaves, pale lavender flowers, and a flattened round fruit that looks like a presliced cake. The leaves and particularly the tough but pliable roots are the parts most often used medicinally. The genus name comes from a Greek word meaning "to heal." Our ancient ancestors billed all mallows as cures for just about any affliction.

Therapeutic Uses:
🍃🍃 Bronchitis, coughing, gastritis, intestinal inflammation, oral inflammation, sore throat.
🍃 Bruises, burns, chafing, chilblains, colds, colitis, Crohn's disease, cystitis, dermatitis, diabetes, gallbladder problems, irritable bowel syndrome, kidney inflammation, respiratory problems, sores, sunburn, ulcers, wounds.
▣ Folk uses: Abscesses, arthritis, asthma, constipation, diarrhea, mucous membrane inflammation, stones, toothache, urethritis, urinary tract infections, varicose veins.

Medicinal Properties:
Marshmallow contains some germ-fighting and inflammation-relieving phytochemicals, as well as compounds that slightly stimulate the immune system. Most of its therapeutic ability, though, arises from large concentrations of mucilage and pectin. Spongy, gummy mucilage soothes and protects inflamed mucous membranes in the throat, stomach, intestines, and urinary tract. Pectin is a soluble fiber that keeps the gastrointestinal system running regularly and helps tame blood sugar. The two substances make a top-notch team for dealing with irritable bowel syndrome and Crohn's disease.

Dosage Options:
One teaspoon of dried leaves or 1 to 2 teaspoons of dried root in a cup of hot water daily, ½ to 1 teaspoon of a liquid root or leaf extract three times a day, ⅛ to ⅓ cup of fresh roots daily, ½ to 2 teaspoons of marshmallow root syrup daily, or 1 teaspoon to 1 tablespoon of marshmallow tincture three times a day. The mucilage becomes gel-like when mixed with a little water; use it as a poultice on inflamed or bruised skin as often as you'd like.

Safety Rating: 2

Precautions:
The high concentration of mucilage and pectin in marshmallow might interfere with or delay absorption of medications, especially if taken simultaneously.

MATÉ *(Ilex paraguariensis)*

What It Is:
Deck the halls with boughs of . . . maté? Yes, the tree whose leaves are used to make a common South American beverage belongs to the holly family. Just like its English kin, the maté tree has bright red berries and shiny leaves. In Paraguay, Argentina, Brazil, and elsewhere across South America, the berries are discarded in favor of the leaves, which are dried, powdered, and used to make a coffeelike pick-me-up.

Therapeutic Uses:
☙☙ Bladder stones, fatigue, irregular heart rhythm, kidney stones, lack of appetite, urinary tract infections.
☙ Asthma, colds, depression, flu, headache, nerve pain, obesity.
▨ Folk use: Arthritis.

Medicinal Properties:
Caffeine gives maté its ability to stimulate the central nervous system and pep you up. (For more information on caffeine's therapeutic qualities, see "Coffee" on page 78.)

Dosage Options:
One teaspoon of maté leaves in a cup of hot water up to three times a day or ½ to 1 teaspoon of a liquid leaf extract one to three times a day.

Safety Rating: 2

Precautions:
Maté is as safe as coffee. (See the precautions under "Coffee" on page 78.)

MEADOWSWEET *(Filipendula ulmaria)*

What It Is:
All plants contain some traces of salicylates, the natural form of aspirin, but several are especially good sources of these compounds. Meadowsweet is one of the better ones. That's why it has long been used to fight colds, flu, fever, arthritis, and achy muscles. Meadowsweet grows in northeastern North America, where it does indeed fill meadows with a sweet fragrance that has been compared to that of almonds. However, the name more likely comes from meadwort, an herb used to flavor mead, a honey-based alcoholic beverage. The plant is a member of the rose family and looks like a low, thorn-free rose.

Therapeutic Uses:
ᴖᴖ Bronchitis, colds, coughing.

ᴖ Acne, arthritis, cellulitis (a deep, spreading tissue inflammation), cervical dysplasia, fever, gout, headache, heart disease, intestinal disease, menstrual pain, muscle pain, peptic ulcers, stomach disease, stones, tissue swelling, toothache, urinary tract infections, water retention.

▨ Folk uses: Bad breath, bruises, congestion, contusions, cramps, cystitis, diarrhea, dizziness, gastric reflux, gravel, heartburn, hematoma, indigestion, kidney disease, labor, liver disease, menstrual excess, mucous membrane inflammation, sprains, ulcers.

Medicinal Properties:
Meadowsweet's salicin resembles that in willow bark, the herb most closely identified with the natural form of aspirin (see "White Willow" on page 221). When acetylsalicylic acid was invented in the late 1800s, manufacturers billed it as easier on your stomach than nature's unacetylated version. That claim may have turned people away from meadowsweet and willow. As it turned out, aspirin proved to be pretty rough on the gut, irritating the stomach and promoting ulcers. In fact, nonsteroidal anti-inflammatory drugs (NSAIDs), of which aspirin is the best known, are responsible for the deaths of 10,000 to 20,000 Americans every year. A lot of herbal experts believe that because of other phytochemicals in the whole herb, meadowsweet (and willow) is actually easier on the stomach than any isolated (or synthesized) salicylate, whether acetylated or not.

Dosage Options:
One to 2 teaspoons of dried flowers steeped in a cup of hot water several times a day, ½ to 1 teaspoon of meadowsweet tincture three times a day, or ½ to 1 teaspoon of a liquid extract up to three times a day.

Safety Rating: 2

Precautions:
If you're allergic to aspirin or have been told by a doctor to avoid aspirin, you probably should not use meadowsweet. Otherwise, the herb is safe, although taking extremely large dosages might make you feel queasy.

MELISSA *(Melissa officinalis)*

See "Lemon Balm" on page 139.

MILK THISTLE *(Silybum marianum)*

What It Is:
Perhaps one of herbal medicine's best-kept secrets and one of American medicine's most glaring oversights, this plant has been used for liver ailments for a couple of thousand years. Native to Europe but now growing along both coasts of North America, milk thistle is an attractive, edible plant with fuzzy, reddish purple flowers. A white veinlike pattern, said in European lore to represent drops of the Virgin Mary's breast milk, decorates its spiny-edged leaves. The markings gave rise to two of the plant's other names, Mary's thistle and holy thistle, and to its folk use as a stimulant of breast milk.

Therapeutic Uses:
🌰🌰 Cirrhosis, colic, gallbladder problems, hepatitis, indigestion, jaundice, lack of appetite, mushroom poisoning.
🌰 Breast cancer, dermatitis, diabetes, diabetic neuropathy, gallstones, high cholesterol, inflammation, intoxication, nausea, obesity, ovarian cancer.
▦ Folk uses: Breast milk deficiency, colic, hemorrhoids, intestinal disease, itching, malaria, menstrual pain, phlebitis, psoriasis, spleen disease, stomach disease, uterine disease.

Medicinal Properties:
Unlike any other synthetic or natural substance known to science, the silymarin in milk thistle (found mostly in its seeds) regenerates liver cells and guards the organ from damage by pollutants, other toxins, and viral invaders. Its ability to lessen the devastation and fatality of cirrhosis, hepatitis, and mushroom poisoning is unparalleled. Studies have shown that silymarin encourages damaged liver cells to regenerate and perform up to par. It deters toxins (whether from alcohol consumption or environmental pollution) from penetrating liver cells. It also guards against free radical oxidation, boosts the body's synthesis of a major antioxidant called glu-

tathione, and lowers fat buildup in the organ (called fatty liver).

A number of studies, most of them conducted in Europe, demonstrate that milk thistle extract extends lives, improves liver function, and relieves symptoms associated with cirrhosis, viral hepatitis, jaundice, and poisoning. It doesn't matter whether the provocation is alcoholism, an overdose of acetaminophen or another drug, overexposure to chemical toxins, or infection by a virus. In one study of people with viral hepatitis, taking 420 milligrams of silymarin for 3 months to a year actually reversed evidence of liver damage, lowered liver enzyme levels, improved blood levels of protein, and lessened symptoms such as fatigue, loss of appetite, and abdominal uneasiness.

Against cirrhosis (which is otherwise essentially untreatable), silymarin averts death and lengthens life. In a comparative experiment of 170 people with cirrhosis that lasted for almost 4 years, 87 people took silymarin every day; the rest ingested a daily placebo that contained nothing of any medicinal importance. In the end, the survival rate for the silymarin takers was 58 percent, as opposed to 39 percent for those in the placebo group. Among silymarin users, 24 died, 18 of them because of liver disease. Among nonusers, 37 died, 31 because of liver complications.

The therapeutic power of silymarin (actually the collective name for a group of four phytochemicals—silybinin, isosilybinin, silydianin, and silychristin) perhaps is best seen in its action against the toxins in poisonous mushrooms, which destroy liver cells. Thousands of people every year get sick or die from ingesting these mushrooms, with almost all the deaths attributed to the death cap mushroom (Amanita phalloides). Studies have shown that animals deliberately poisoned with these mushrooms do not die if they also ingest silymarin. In other studies, survival rates increased for people who inadvertently ingested death caps but were then given experimental dosages of milk thistle's phytochemicals.

Prescription Counterparts:
There are no pharmaceutical alternatives to milk thistle for treating cirrhosis or mushroom poisoning. For hepatitis C, mainstream medicine uses injections of the anticancer, antiviral drug interferon (Roferon-A). The medication doesn't have a very high success rate, and it is costly and fraught with side effects.

Dosage Options:
A standardized supplement providing 70 to 80 percent (or 420 to 840 milligrams) of silymarin daily, 1 teaspoon of mashed milk thistle seeds in a cup of hot water an hour or so before meals, 1 to 2 teaspoons of a liquid extract daily, or up to 1,070 milligrams of milk thistle capsules daily. You can also munch on the seeds as you would sunflower seeds. The roots and leaves (trimmed of their prickly points) may be eaten either raw or cooked. Young flower buds can be cooked and eaten.

Safety Rating: 3

Precautions:
None reported, even in large doses, except for isolated cases of an upset stomach or diarrhea.

MISTLETOE *(Viscum album)*

What It Is:
To the Druids, mistletoe was magical. It needs no contact with soil to survive and thrive, appearing spontaneously and growing entirely in trees. We now know there's no magic involved; instead, this is a case of plant parasitism. Mistletoe's seeds, spread from tree to tree by birds, sprout small roots that puncture branches and take hold. Sprigs of the plant—with its thick oval leaves, clusters of light yellow or green flowers, and white berries—used to be hung in homes to ward off bad luck, witches, and illness. This practice eventually gave rise to the tradition of hanging mistletoe above a doorway during the Christmas season. You would do well to keep this poisonous plant there; ingesting it can be the kiss of death.

Therapeutic Uses:
～～ Arthritis, tumors.
～ Inflammation, neuroses, sores.
▦ Folk uses: Abscesses, anxiety, asthma, cancer, chorea (involuntary spasms of the face and limbs), diarrhea, dizziness, epilepsy, fatigue, gout, hardening of the arteries, headache, hemorrhage, high blood pressure, hysteria, lack of menstruation, nervousness, rapid heart rate.

Medicinal Properties:
Mistletoe has been widely studied in Europe, principally because of a patented drug made from the plant's fermented juices. The injectable serum, called Iscador, accelerates immune system activity and speeds white blood cells to attack and cordon off tumors. The medication has been tested on people against cancers of the breast, cervix, colon, lungs, and stomach, and some slight improvement has been shown. Some American alternative physicians also have access to injectable mistletoe from Europe and incorporate it into their cancer treatments, but the FDA has not authorized its use.

Dosage Options:
No amount in any supplemental form is safe (see "Precautions"). If you choose to take mistletoe, do so only under the direction of an herb-savvy physician.

Safety Rating:
Do not use.

Precautions:
Mistletoe, both its leaves and especially its berries, is toxic, with a definite lethal potential. At the least, it can cause hepatitis, low blood pressure, seizures, pupil dilation, and coma. At the worst, it can cause either immediate death from respiratory failure or death after a few days from wasting away. The controversial clinical injections used in Europe and experimentally by some American alternative physicians can cause allergic reactions, chest pains, chills, circulatory difficulties, fever, and

headaches. Iscador should be viewed as a toxic prescription-only pharmaceutical to be used only by physicians versed in its effects.

MOTHERWORT *(Leonurus cardiaca)*

What It Is:
The botanical name gives away the plant's traditional and current use. Motherwort has been used for hundreds of years in Europe and China for all manner of heart problems and circulatory disorders. The perennial, native to Europe and naturalized across much of North America, features a tall single stem from which grow three-fingered leaves in an arrangement said to resemble a lion's tail, the source of another common name. Clusters of prickly, pinkish white flowers grow close to the stem.

Therapeutic Uses:
ᴥᴥ Heart disease, hyperthyroidism (Graves' disease), irregular heart rhythm.
ᴥ Cramps, high blood pressure, insomnia, neuroses, rapid heart rate, stroke.
▨ Folk uses: Anxiety, asthma, fatigue, fever, gas, labor, lack of menstruation, menstrual pain, neuralgia, palpitations, sciatica, stomachache.

Medicinal Properties:
Science endorses motherwort's folk applications against heart-related conditions. Chinese research shows that it promotes a better volume of blood throughout the body and can slow a rapid heart rate. Some of its phytochemicals can help relax you and relieve stress, which also may contribute to its cardiac qualities.

Dosage Options:
One to 2 teaspoons of the dried herb in a cup of water once or twice a day, ½ to 1 teaspoon of a liquid extract up to three times a day, or ½ to 1 teaspoon of motherwort tincture three times a day.

Safety Rating: 2

Precautions:
None reported. Avoid its use if you're pregnant or nursing. Dosages larger than 3 grams might cause diarrhea, indigestion, or uterine bleeding. A few particularly sensitive people might get a skin reaction upon contact with the plant.

MUIRA PUAMA *(Ptychopetalum olacoides)*

What It Is:
A large, rather nondescript tree with simple, untoothed evergreen leaves, muira puama, like thousands of other tropical species, enjoys little recognition outside the Amazonian rain forest. North Americans might know it by another name, potency wood.

Therapeutic Uses:
 Folk uses: Arthritis, diarrhea, erectile dysfunction, hookworm, indigestion, lack of appetite, lack of menstruation, low libido, pain, poliomyelitis.

Medicinal Properties:
Muira puama has gone virtually unexamined in scientific circles, but it has a long reputation in South America as an aphrodisiac and nerve stimulant. One clinical study endorsed its use for rekindling desire and restoring erectile ability. After 262 men took a muira puama extract for 2 weeks, 62 percent of those with low libido reported a revived interest in sex, and 51 percent of those with erectile dysfunction claimed that the herb provided at least some benefit.

Prescription Counterparts:
Muira puama deserves a try before you ask your doctor for sildenafil citrate (Viagra). It might work for you, and it's certainly cheaper than the pharmaceutical.

Dosage Options:
One-half to 1¼ teaspoons of a liquid root extract or 1 dropper of a tincture about 30 minutes before sexual activity.

Safety Rating: 1

Precautions:
None reported.

MULLEIN *(Verbascum, various species)*

What It Is:
Another common name for this towering biennial, flannel leaf, is a tip-off to how the plant looks and feels. Its big tobacco-like leaves, stalk, and little yellow flowers, which sprout from the top of the stem, all are coated with a flannel-like down. Just as you might don a flannel shirt to stay warm, old-timers used to line their shoes with mullein leaves to keep out winter cold. Indigenous to Europe but naturalized in various parts of North America, mullein also is said to prevent colds and breathing ailments of all kinds. Smoking the dried leaves was a common folk remedy for

congestion and respiratory infections. Traditionally, a yellow dye made from its flowers was used as a hair rinse, and women once rubbed its leaves on their cheeks instead of applying rouge.

Therapeutic Uses:

～～ Bronchitis, coughing, mucous membrane inflammation.

～ Colds, congestion, dermatitis, diarrhea, hemorrhoids, inflammation, intestinal disease, respiratory disease, sore throat, tuberculosis, wounds.

▨ Folk uses: Asthma, cramps, earache, ear inflammation, fever, kidney disease, migraine, pain, sores, tumors.

Medicinal Properties:

The silky, milky mucilage in mullein leaves underlies its ability to soothe inflamed mucous membranes, although little scientific study backs this up. Saponins in the plant may account for its folk reputation as an expectorant that breaks up congestion.

Dosage Options:

One-half to 1 teaspoon of a liquid extract daily, 3 to 4 teaspoons of dried or fresh mullein flowers in a cup of hot water once or twice a day, 1 to 2 tablespoons of fresh leaves daily, or ¼ to 1 teaspoon of a tincture three or four times a day. Don't honor the tradition of smoking dried mullein leaves.

Safety Rating: 2

Precautions:

None reported.

MYRRH *(Commiphora myrrha)*

What It Is:
Some botanical authorities say that the three wise men carried myrrh not to bestow a gift on the Christ child but to treat canker sores they might develop along the way. The gummy resin that flows from this almost leafless Middle Eastern shrub is an ancient remedy for mouth sores, as well as a very pleasant incense. Other people speculate that the wise men actually bore a similar resin called gugul, whose native India is a long way from the Holy Land. Even among experts, the two plants are almost indistinguishable. (For more information on this question, see "Gugul" on page 122 and "Boswellia" on page 51.)

Therapeutic Uses:
ᴖᴖ Oral inflammation, sore throat.

ᴖ Abrasions, asthma, athlete's foot, bronchial disease, canker sores, colds, congestion, dandruff and other scaly skin conditions, dermatitis, diabetes, gingivitis, oral ulcers, sinusitis, sores, tonsillitis.

▦ Folk uses: Bedsores, boils, cancer, diabetes, gas, hemorrhoids, hoarseness, indigestion, leprosy, mucous membrane inflammation, nasal disease, stomach disease, swelling, ulcers, wounds.

Medicinal Properties:
Most plants contain antibacterial phytochemicals, and folklore suggests that myrrh does, too. Other than that, given the complexities of this plant family and the dearth of taxonomic information, it's difficult to enumerate with certainty myrrh's medicinal qualities. The gums from some *Commiphora* species, like many other gums, have displayed an ability to keep blood running freely, lower cholesterol and triglycerides, protect the heart, and guard against oxidation (see "Gugul" on page 122).

Dosage Options:
One teaspoon of powdered myrrh in a cup of hot water once or twice a day, 8 to 10 drops of myrrh extract up to four times a day, 1 gram of myrrh resin three times a day, ½ to 1 teaspoon of myrrh tincture daily, or 5 to 10 drops of the tincture in a glass of water as a gargle or mouthwash as often as desired.

Safety Rating: 2

Precautions:
None reported in recognized dosages. Taking as much as 2 to 4 grams could cause diarrhea or kidney inflammation. People with diabetes should take extra care if using myrrh; it may contribute to the sugar-lowering effect of insulin and other hypoglycemic drugs. Pregnant women, nursing mothers, and those prone to uterine bleeding also should be on the lookout. Especially sensitive people might experience burning or irritation if undiluted myrrh tincture is applied topically. Other sensitive people might get the hiccups or feel somewhat restless.

NEEM *(Azadirachta indica)*

What It Is:
Some organic gardeners, whether they know it or not, are big neem users. A number of natural, nontoxic pesticides (which smell somewhat like garlic) contain leaf or seed oils from this tree, which is oaklike in stature but actually a member of the mahogany family. Though native to India, neem now grows freely in many subtropical areas, including Florida, southern California, and Southeast Asia. It's extensively cultivated in arid lands for its ability to free up some nutrients from infertile soils.

Therapeutic Uses:
Dermatitis, diabetes, fever, gingivitis, heart disease, inflammation, malaria, pain, plaque, scabies, ulcers, worms, wounds.
Folk use: Hemorrhoids.

Medicinal Properties:
As folk medicine and modern science attest, neem vanquishes vermin. Preparations of the plant have long been used against insect infestations and personal invasions, including intestinal worms, malaria, scabies, and lice. In a study of people with scabies, a parasitic skin infection by mites, 98 percent of the participants were cured with topical preparations of neem and turmeric. The tree also helps kill bacteria and fungi, and extracts are included in some commercially available toothpastes (check the labels).

Dosage Options:
Two to four 500-milligram capsules containing neem leaf powder with meals.

Safety Rating: 1

Precautions:
Among adults, no problems reported in recommended amounts, although excessive dosages could cause breathing difficulties, convulsions, stupor, and even death. Infants and children should not take the herb at all. For reasons not yet understood, neem's oils appear to be more toxic to youngsters than to grown-ups.

NETTLE *(Urtica dioica)*

What It Is:
Have you urticated yourself today? People have been doing it for a couple of thousand years to relieve arthritis pain, hives, rashes, and even sciatica. To perform urtication, all you need is a nettle plant and a glove. Put on the glove, pick up the plant, and smack yourself repeatedly. Far-fetched as it may seem, urtication, a term based on nettle's botanical name, frequently works pretty well. From its stiff stem to its jagged-edged, heart-shaped leaves, the plant is blanketed with small fuzzy hairs, hence one of its common names, stinging nettle. Part of the treatment's success is that the little hairs serve as a counterirritant, but some phytomedicine also is being injected into your skin. Nettle is native to Europe and Asia, but it's now found across southern Canada and most of the United States. Its medicinal applications haven't been limited to self-flagellation. Australians and others are longtime advocates of nettle tea and nettle root juice to open up bronchial passages.

Therapeutic Uses:
~~ Arthritis, bladder stones, gravel, hay fever, kidney stones, prostate enlargement (benign), prostatitis, urinary pain or problems, urinary tract infections.

~ Allergies, asthma, bed-wetting, bronchitis, bug bites, burns, consumption, dermatitis, diarrhea, dysentery, fever, goiter, gout, hemorrhage, hives and other skin eruptions, nosebleeds, oral inflammation, osteoarthritis, osteoporosis, rhinitis, sciatica.

▒ Folk uses: Ague, anemia, cancer, colitis, congestion, eczema, gallbladder problems, hair loss, hemorrhoids, jaundice, kidney disease, labor, menstrual pain, nerve pain, sore throat, spleen enlargement, sprains, tendinitis, urethral bleeding, vaginitis, wounds.

Medicinal Properties:
Science says there's medicine in the madness of urtication. Stinging nettle contains natural antihistamines and anti-inflammatories (including quercetin) that open up constricted bronchial and nasal passages, making it a choice therapy for treating asthma and nasal allergies. Some herbal authorities assert that no other natural remedy eases hay fever symptoms so markedly. The anti-inflammatory substances join with rich concentrations of the minerals boron and silicon to help ease the pain of rheumatoid arthritis and osteoarthritis, as well as tendinitis and bursitis. Boron also helps our bones retain calcium, so it should come as no surprise that nettle has shown some benefit against osteoporosis.

Extracts of nettle roots are reliable diuretics that encourage excretion, especially of uric acid, but simultaneously discourage nighttime urges to go to the bathroom. This somewhat unusual dichotomy makes stinging nettle a notable help against such disparate problems as gout, bed-wetting, and, as one small study demonstrated, the overnight urinary woes of benign prostate enlargement. Concerning the latter, certain compounds appear to deter a key chemical process involved in prostate enlargement—the conversion of testosterone into a form that forces the gland to grow. Urination stimulation also helps treat kidney stones, bladder stones, and urinary tract infections.

Prescription Counterparts:
Before you shell out the cash for finasteride (Proscar) to treat benign prostate enlargement, consider combining stinging nettle with saw palmetto and pumpkin (see "Saw Palmetto" on page 195 and "Pumpkin" on page 179). Together, these foods are at least as effective as the synthetic drug, and they certainly don't pose the same threat of erection-killing side effects.

Dosage Options:
One 450-milligram standardized supplement twice a day, 3 to 4 teaspoons of dried nettle leaves in a cup of boiling water up to four times a day, ½ to 1 teaspoon of a liquid herb extract or root tincture three times a day, or up to 1 tablespoon of an herb tincture daily. You can also eat fresh nettle leaves as a vegetable. Steaming and drying removes the sting. The remaining "pot liquor," by the way, is a good therapeutic tea.

Safety Rating: 3

Precautions:
For the herb, none reported. For root preparations, a sensitive person might experience mild gastric upset or a skin reaction. Urtication is not recommended, but if you try it, remember to put on a glove before picking up the hairy plant. Depending on how hard you swat yourself, the stinging can be painful and irritating for at least several minutes. Some people may even wind up getting black-and-blue marks.

OATS *(Avena sativa)*

What It Is:
Oats certainly deserve their reputation as a wholesome, healthful, nourishing food. They're easy to digest, soothing to an irritated throat, and loaded with soluble fiber to keep the intestinal tract running regularly. In the 1800s, doctors advocated oat straw as a nerve tonic, good for nervous exhaustion and debility. After its introduction from Europe, oat grass came to be cultivated all over North America and now often grows wild.

Therapeutic Uses:
🌿🌿 Dermatitis, high cholesterol, inflammation, itching, seborrhea, warts.
🌿 Constipation, osteoporosis, sore throat.
▦ Folk uses: Addiction, anxiety, arthritis, colitis, coughing, debility, depression, diabetes, diarrhea, eczema, eye inflammation, fatigue, flu, frostbite, gallbladder problems, gout, hardening of the arteries, heart disease, high triglycerides, impetigo, insomnia, intestinal disease, kidney disease, liver disease, menstrual pain, morphine addiction, neurasthenia, nicotine addiction, poison ivy, stomach disease, stress, urinary tract infections.

Medicinal Properties:
Phytochemicals called beta-glucans are responsible for oats' well-advertised help in lowering cholesterol, although they aren't the best source of these phytochemicals (barley is better). Oats aren't the best source of soluble fiber either (barley is better in this case, too). But oats are good "food farmacy." The green tops of the plant are rich in silica, which encourages excretion of gout-causing uric acid. Applied topically, oatmeal is quite good for relieving the itch of psoriasis, scabies, and other skin conditions. Finally, eating the wild grass might just buck up the libido.

Dosage Options:
Eat oats as often as you can. Supplement suggestions include ½ to 1 teaspoon of a liquid oat seed extract daily, ½ to 1 teaspoon of oat tincture three times a day, 1 tablespoon of oats in a cup of hot water every day, or 1 to 2 tablespoons of the fresh herb daily. You can also dump about 4 ounces of dry oats into your bathwater or whip up a batch of oatmeal, put it in some cheesecloth, and apply it to your itchy skin.

Safety Rating: 3

Precautions:
None reported. Even most people with celiac disease or a sensitivity to gluten can eat oats.

OLIVE LEAF *(Olea europea)*

What It Is:
The monounsaturated oil of this evergreen's fruit is the star attraction of the heart-protecting Mediterranean diet. The olive has been grown in Egypt, Israel, and Syria since biblical times but is now cultivated across the Mediterranean region, as well as in Peru, Chile, and elsewhere in South America. Amid the monounsaturated mania, the rest of the tree has gotten short shrift until recently. Its slender, feather-shaped leaves—pale green on top, almost silver on the flip side, and about 2 inches long—may be coming into their own medicinally.

Therapeutic Uses:
☙ Bacterial infections, diabetes, fungal infections, gout, heart disease, high blood pressure.
▓ Folk uses: Fever, wounds.

Medicinal Properties:
In folk medicine, olive leaves were used to disinfect wounds. Toward the end of the nineteenth century, scientists discovered a phytochemical in the leaves called oleuropein, which appears to kill bacteria and fungi. The extract, which also fights off free radical oxidation, has gained some popularity as a treatment for colds and infections. Herbal authorities, though, are by no means in agreement on this; just because an isolated extract may do something doesn't mean that the whole herb will. In other research, in Japan, olive leaves increased urinary output and lowered uric acid levels, both a big help to people with gout.

Dosage Options:
Put 2 teaspoons of dried olive leaves in a cup of hot water and steep for 30 minutes before drinking. (Participants in the Japanese study cited above ingested 4 cups of olive leaf tea daily for 3 weeks.) For a supplement, 500 milligrams of an olive leaf powdered extract standardized for 6 percent oleuropein daily. Otherwise, follow the dosage suggestions on the product's label.

Safety Rating: 2

Precautions:
None reported in recommended dosages. Some observers say that olive leaves might upset your intestinal tract if taken on an empty stomach.

ONION *(Allium cepa)*

What It Is:
Onion is garlic's teary-eyed sibling in the *Allium* genus. Both grow below ground, and both shoot thin green leaves above the earth. Onion, however, sprouts round leaves and a tall central stem that's topped by a round cluster of tiny, greenish white flowers. It isn't quite as pungent as its kin and may be more agreeable to sensitive stomachs.

Therapeutic Uses:
🖎🖎 Bronchitis, colds, coughing, diabetes, fever, hardening of the arteries, high blood pressure, high cholesterol, immune system problems, indigestion, infections, inflammation, inflammatory bowel disease, lack of appetite, oral inflammation, sore throat.

🖎 Asthma, cancer, congestion, earache, heart disease, high triglycerides, osteoporosis, stomachache, stomach cancer, yeast infections.

▦ Folk uses: Acne, boils, bruises, bug bites, burns, chest pain, cholera, colic, ear inflammation, jaundice, menstrual pain, sores, warts, whooping cough, wounds.

Medicinal Properties:
Onion shares, albeit in somewhat smaller amounts, many of garlic's phytochemicals, particularly alliin and other sulfur compounds. It also shares the same therapeutic potential, notably against heart disease, high cholesterol, high blood pressure, infections, and pain. For instance, for half of the people with moderately high cholesterol in one study, taking 2 to 3 tablespoons of onion oil daily reduced blood fat levels by 7 to 33 percent. The newest research suggests that onion also might be useful against osteoporosis. (For more on this family's medicinal possibilities, see "Garlic" on page 106.)

Onion outshines garlic in its use against diabetes, asthma, allergies, and other inflammatory respiratory conditions. This is because of onion's high quercetin content, much of which resides in the skin. This bioflavonoid fights allergies, tames the body's inflammation-generating responses (it's excellent for inflammatory bowel disease), protects capillaries from harm, helps tame high blood sugar, and perhaps interferes with the formation of cataracts.

Dosage Options:
When cooking onions, don't remove the skins; that's where most of the quercetin is concentrated. Instead, filter the skins out of soups and other foods before eating. In supplement form, 1 teaspoon of onion juice three or four times a day, 4 to 5 teaspoons of onion tincture daily, or 4 to 5 tablespoons of onion syrup daily.

Safety Rating: 3

Precautions:
None reported, except for a few rare instances of allergic reactions.

OREGON GRAPE *(Mahonia aquifolia)*

What It Is:
A strange, attractive evergreen planted as an ornamental, Oregon grape (also known as mountain grape) is a hardy shrub indigenous to the western United States. It has a yellowish inner bark, yellowish flowers, and purple, grape-shaped edible fruit. This fruit, which is well-protected by sharp-toothed leaves that look like holly leaves, is sometimes used to make wine and brandy. Oregon grape shares many phytochemicals with goldenseal, goldthread, barberry, and yellowroot, even though not all are botanically related.

Therapeutic Uses:
❧ Dandruff, dermatitis, psoriasis.
▨ Folk uses: Acne, bruises, constipation, coughing, eczema, jaundice, kidney disease, liver disease, stones, ulcers, urinary tract infections, wounds.

Medicinal Properties:
For most health-related applications, consider Oregon grape an acceptable substitute for goldenseal (see "Goldenseal" on page 117). Both contain many of the same phytochemical compounds, including the immune-stimulating, infection-fighting, virus-killing antiseptic berberine. Goldenseal, which is currently an endangered species, may be better known among herb aficionados, but it's not necessarily better for all indications. Aside from its berberine, Oregon grape is also a muscular antioxidant and contains substances that help deter the formation of certain skin cells, which is why it's useful against psoriasis and other dermatologic conditions.

Prescription Counterparts:
Natural berberine performs well against its pharmaceutical competition (see "Goldenseal" on page 117).

Dosage Options:
One-quarter to ½ teaspoon of a liquid root extract daily or ½ teaspoon of dried root or bark in a cup of hot water once a day.

Safety Rating: 1

Precautions:
Probably not for long-term use (see the precautions under "Goldenseal" on page 117). Consult a qualified physician.

PAPAYA *(Carica papaya)*

What It Is:
When you drink a beer, chances are you're imbibing a little bit of papain from this exotic fruit. That proteolytic (protein-digesting) enzyme breaks up particulates in the brew, allowing it to remain clear once it's chilled.

Native to Central and South America but found in tropical climates around the world, papaya plants serve many purposes. The bark is good for making rope. The long leaves turn tough meat into a tenderized treat and serve as a stain-removing soap substitute. The yellowish orange fruit—which may be egg-shaped, pear-shaped, or football-shaped, with a corresponding diversity in length—make great juices, breakfast foods, jellies, and preserves. The milklike juice from unripe fruit, called latex, contains the most concentration of papain—enough, some people say, to remove freckles.

Therapeutic Uses:
🐛 Blood clots, disc inflammation, heartburn, indigestion, infertility, ringworm, worms.
▦ Folk uses: Abscesses, arthritis, blood clots, bronchitis, burns, circulatory problems, constipation, depression, enlarged lymph glands, eye inflammation, flu, freckles, gallbladder problems, gas, hardening of the arteries, heart disease, hematoma, hemorrhoids, Hodgkin's disease, infections, infertility, inflammation, intestinal disease, lack of appetite, leukemia, liver disease, lymphoma, nerve inflammation, neurasthenia, oral inflammation, pancreatic inflammation, parasitic infections, phlebitis, psoriasis, rectal disease, respiratory disease, sore throat, stomach disease, tissue swelling, tumors, ulcers, urethritis, uterine inflammation, vaginal disease, varicose veins, water retention, wounds, yeast infections.

Medicinal Properties:
Papain's protein-digesting power makes papaya helpful against heartburn and indigestion. Mixed with a little honey and taken before meals, it may even prevent heartburn. Papain also may help thin the blood and discourage clotting. The fruit's proteolytic enzymes and other compounds, including a substance called carpaine, work against intestinal worms and other parasites. Some experiments conducted on lab rats suggest that papaya seeds might reverse infertility.

Prescription Counterparts:

Some research indicates that papain can magnify the blood-thinning action of the pharmaceutical warfarin (Coumadin). If you're taking warfarin, don't shy away from papaya. Instead, talk to an herb-savvy physician to see if you can rely on smaller dosages of the drug. Back in 1988, the FDA authorized doctors to use injections of chymopapain, another papaya enzyme, to help break up protein complexes involved in slipped discs.

Dosage Options:

Ten to 50 milligrams of papain, 1 to 3 teaspoons of papaya juice, 1 to 2 teaspoons of dried papaya leaves in a cup of hot water, 1 to 2 tablespoons of the fresh fruit, or ½ to 1 teaspoon of elixir of papaya daily. For help against intestinal worms and other parasites, munch on a dozen or so papaya seeds. Be forewarned, though: They're almost as hot as mustard seeds.

Safety Rating: 3

Precautions:

None reported for papaya leaves. Excessive consumption of the fruit might cause a perforated esophagus. Papain might enhance the blood-thinning action of the drug warfarin. Ingesting too much papain could cause stomach inflammation. Applied externally, it might cause dermatitis in some sensitive people.

PARSLEY *(Petroselinum crispum)*

What It Is:

Parsley is a perennial . . . table scrap. According to some estimates, at least 90 percent of all parsley sprigs used to garnish restaurant meals are left untouched and tossed in the trash. Diners apparently prefer the breath mints often available next to the cash register to nature's own breath of fresh air. This disrespect is a far cry from the days of ancient Greece, when athletes were adorned with parsley crowns and tombs were decorated with parsley wreaths. Back then, the herb was too revered to be put on a plate and eaten. Since then, this carrot-family member has become a familiar flavoring in soups, sauces, and stews, not to mention a nearly ubiquitous garnish.

Therapeutic Uses:

🌿🌿 Bladder stones, gravel, kidney stones, urinary pain or problems, urinary tract infections.

🌿 Bad breath, breast milk deficiency, colic, gallstones, indigestion, low libido (in women), menstrual pain, osteoporosis.

▨ Folk uses: Arthritis, asthma, black-and-blue marks, breast tenderness, bronchitis, bruises, colds, congestion, coughing, cystitis, dropsy, hair loss, heart disease, high blood pressure, infections, intestinal inflammation, jaundice, kidney disease, labor, lack of menstruation, lice, liver disease, muscle pain, skin problems, spleen disorders, stomachache, tumors.

Medicinal Properties:
The chlorophyll in parsley is a mighty mediator of bad breath, but that's not all this plant has to offer. Parsley stimulates urination, making it a good adjunct to any therapy for breast tenderness, kidney stones, bladder stones, gravel, urinary infections, and urinary difficulties. The folkloric use against menstrual and other female-specific problems may have some scientific basis: The herb's phytochemicals are mildly estrogenic. Its high concentrations of boron and fluoride might help against bone thinning and osteoporosis. Parsley also helps inhibit the body's release of histamines, which is perhaps why naturopathic healers prescribe it for colds and congestion.

Dosage Options:
Chew on a sprig or two after every meal. Other options include 1 to 2 teaspoons of dried parsley leaves or roots in a cup of hot water daily, 1 teaspoon of bruised seeds in a cup of hot water daily, ½ to 1 teaspoon of a liquid extract three times a day, 2 to 4 tablespoons of the fresh herb daily, or ½ to 1 teaspoon of a liquid seed or root extract daily. With frequent topical applications, black-and-blue marks often vanish in a day or so.

Safety Rating: 3

Precautions:
As a food, parsley rarely, if ever, poses a problem. Some herbal analysts caution against ingesting extracts and other concentrated forms if you have kidney inflammation or are pregnant. People with particularly sensitive skin could become more sensitive to sunlight. The herb also may increase the action of prescription monoamine oxidase inhibitors (MAOIs). The myristicin in parsley can, in a sufficiently high concentration that you're unlikely to ingest, impair hearing, slow the pulse rate, lower blood pressure, damage the liver, and cause other reactions.

PARTRIDGEBERRY *(Mitchella repens)*

What It Is:
With its round, shiny, white-streaked leaves, white flowers, and bright red berries, partridgeberry often decorates rock gardens and lawns. But this ground-hugging evergreen, native to North America, has more than ornamental value. For a clue to its medicinal worth and who initially used it, consider another of the plant's common names: squaw vine.

Therapeutic Uses:

🍃 Inflammation.

🔲 Folk uses: Arthritis, breast milk deficiency, dysentery, hemorrhoids, hives, labor, lack of menstruation, menstrual pain, pain.

Medicinal Properties:

Native American women considered partridgeberry one of the best natural treatments for many uniquely female health problems—from easing menstrual cramps and stimulating regular menstruation to facilitating childbirth and soothing nipple soreness from nursing. Herbalists who specialize in women's concerns generally agree, continuing to recommend partridgeberry tea in the final few weeks of pregnancy and a salve made from the plant to alleviate nipple soreness.

Dosage Options:

One-half to 1 teaspoon of a liquid extract daily. For nipple soreness, apply the extract topically as needed.

Safety Rating: 2

Precautions:

None reported.

PASSIONFLOWER *(Passiflora incarnata)*

What It Is:

Spanish explorers in North America believed that this vine's pale lavender flowers, from the corona and stamens to the number of petals, represented many aspects of the Crucifixion, or Passion, of Christ. Native Americans cherished it for other reasons, using its three-fingered leaves to speed the healing of bruises. Later herbal physicians realized that it calms nervous tension and is mildly sedating.

Therapeutic Uses:

🍃🍃 Insomnia, menstrual pain, nervousness, restlessness.

🍃 Earache, epilepsy, headache, hemorrhoids, high blood pressure, hyperactivity, hysteria, infections, nerve pain, rapid heart rate, stress, yeast infections.

🔲 Folk uses: Addiction, anxiety, asthma, boils, bruises, colic, cramps, cuts, depression, diarrhea, gastritis, heart disease, intestinal inflammation, muscle pain, palpitations.

Medicinal Properties:

Picking apart a plant chemically often isn't a useful exercise, for the whole extract usually is more effective (and safer) than any individual constituent. This is especially so for passionflower. Together in an extract, the alkaloids and flavonoids are stronger sedatives and relaxants than any one on its own. Nevertheless, we do know that harmine and harmaline induce drowsiness, ease smooth-muscle cramps, and, as some prescription antidepressants do, curb the body's release of the monoamine oxidase (MAO) enzyme. Apigenin and other flavonoids relax, reduce anxiety, stop spasms, and soothe inflammation. The phytochemical passicol fights a number of bacteria, molds, and yeasts. The herb also shows some ability to lessen postherpes nerve pain.

Prescription Counterparts:
At one time, the FDA okayed passionflower for inclusion in nonprescription insomnia remedies, but in the late 1970s, it withdrew its support for lack of evidence supporting the herb's effectiveness. Tell that to users of over-the-counter sleep aids in Great Britain and Germany, where American passionflower is widely used. The herb might help lessen your reliance on pharmaceutical benzodiazepines such as diazepam (Valium) and chlordiazepoxide hydrochloride (Librium).

Dosage Options:
One hundred fifty to 300 milligrams of a solid leaf extract daily, ⅛ to ¼ teaspoon of a liquid leaf or whole-herb extract three times a day, ½ to 1 teaspoon of passionflower tincture daily, or 1 teaspoon of dried flowers in a cup of hot water up to three times a day.

Safety Rating: 2

Precautions:
None reported with prudent use. Extremely large doses may depress the central nervous system or enhance the effects of any monoamine oxidase (MAOs) inhibitors you may be taking for depression. Then again, you're not even supposed to eat cheese or drink wine if you're on those antidepressants. In lab animals, at least, harmine and harmaline stimulate uterine contractions. If you're pregnant, you may want to think twice before taking this herb.

PAU D'ARCO (*Tabebuia*, various species)

What It Is:
In the Brazilian variation of Portuguese, *pau d'arco* translates as "bow tree." This is just one name (*ipe roxo, tahibo,* and *tahuari* are others) for a medicinally important genus that grows in savannas and rain forests. Some species have pink or purple flowers; others have yellow blooms. Many even flower during the dry season, when the trees are leafless. The wood of some species is so hard that it'll damage an ax head.

Therapeutic Uses:
🌿 Athlete's foot, cancer, dermatitis, eczema, Epstein-Barr virus, infections, leukemia, malaria, schistosomiasis, skin cancer, ulcers, vaginal inflammation, wounds, yeast infections.

⊞ Folk uses: Anemia, arthritis, dysentery, fungal infections, hemorrhoids, Hodgkin's disease, immune system problems, psoriasis, scabies, sore throat.

Medicinal Properties:
In Brazil and elsewhere across South America and the world, pau d'arco bark is an accepted remedy for vaginal yeast infections, other fungal infections, immune system weakness, and cancer. Extracts of the whole herb do appear to fight yeast and fungal infections, and early investigations displayed some promise against malignancies. But isolated formulations of two phytochemicals, lapachol and beta-lapachone, proved to be otherwise toxic in amounts necessary to kill cancer cells. Low doses of the isolated phytochemicals activate the body's immune system, but higher amounts suppress it. Herbal authorities cite these findings as more proof that extracts of the whole herb are better than any isolated compound. The bottom line is that pau d'arco seems to be more promising as an herbal remedy for fungal woes than malignant cancers.

Prescription Counterparts:
The lapachol and beta-lapachone in pau d'arco have been compared favorably to the yeast-killing drug ketoconazole (Nizoral). Some say that beta-lapachone is better than the pharmaceutical.

Dosage Options:
Three hundred to 1,500 milligrams of dried pau d'arco bark in divided doses over the course of a day, ½ to 1 teaspoon or so of a liquid extract, 15 to 20 grams of ground bark in a pint of water, or ¼ to ½ cup of fresh inner bark daily.

Safety Rating: 1

Precautions:
Supplements and other preparations of the whole bark present no known threat of serious side effects, although some people might get nauseous. Isolated lapachol and beta-lapachone do pose grim risks. Studies show that ingesting 500 milligrams of pure lapachol for every 2.2 pounds of body weight is lethal. Taking six doses of just 9 milligrams of pure beta-lapachone caused diarrhea, weight loss, and ultimately death.

PEPPERMINT *(Mentha x piperita)*

What It Is:
Almost from the moment the first Roman munched on a mint leaf after dining, a postprandial tradition was born. It wasn't until the late 1600s, though, that the prescriptive possibilities behind the cool taste began to be acknowledged. Peppermint is now probably the most widely used of all volatile essential oils, found in every-

thing from laxatives, antacids, salves, and cold nostrums to toothpastes, mouth-washes, and after-dinner candy. Some two dozen species, with hundreds of vari-eties, populate the genus *Mentha*, including spearmint and European pennyroyal, but peppermint is a better source of menthol than either of these two. The plant is actually a hybrid of spearmint and watermint; all three are native to Europe but are now grown the world over. There are several varieties of peppermint, each with its own unique traits, but they all generally sport purplish white flowers and jagged-edged oval leaves on short leaf stalks.

Therapeutic Uses:

🌿🌿 Breathing difficulties, colitis, gallbladder disease, gastritis, infections, intestinal inflammation, irritable bowel syndrome, lack of appetite, liver disease, mucous membrane inflammation, muscle pain, nerve pain, oral inflammation, sore throat.

🌿 Arthritis, asthma, bile blockage, bronchitis, bug bites, colds, cold sores, colic, congestion, coughing, cramps, fever, flu, gas, headache, hemorrhoids, herpes, indi-gestion, itching, nausea, neuroses, pain, sinusitis, stomachache, tendinitis, toothache.

▨ Folk uses: Flu, gingivitis, heartburn, insomnia, menstrual pain, morning sick-ness, motion sickness, pneumonia, stress.

Medicinal Properties:

Most of the mints' medicine is in the menthol, concentrated primarily in pepper-mint's volatile essential oil. The phytochemical does far more than freshen the breath, however. It tames smooth-muscle spasms in the intestinal tract, relaxes tight skeletal muscles, improves the flow of bile and aids in breaking up gallstones, thins mucus, kills certain bacteria and viruses, and helps deaden pain. Other com-pounds also help break up congestion. Clinical studies have verified the herb's abil-ity to quell intestinal muscle spasms and ease irritable bowel symptoms. Other long-term experiments have shown that menthol, along with related peppermint phytochemicals, helps dissolve gallstones without the need for surgery.

Prescription Counterparts:

Peppermint is a worthy competitor to the various pharmaceuticals prescribed for irritable bowel syndrome and other intestinal problems, and it doesn't pose the same risks as those drugs. For instance, Librax, a combination of the sedative chlor-diazepoxide hydrochloride (Librium) and the antispasmodic clidinium bromide (Quarzan), can cause drowsiness, confusion, constipation, nausea, water retention, tissue swelling, jaundice, and blurred vision. It also may contribute to glaucoma and prostate enlargement. All that and the drug is deemed only "possibly effective" against irritable bowel syndrome and peptic ulcers. Donnatal, which combines phe-nobarbital with atropine and other unsavory pharmaceuticals, also is only "possibly effective." It may magnify the risk of glaucoma or urinary tract difficulties; compli-cate problems associated with liver and kidney disorders, an overactive thyroid, heart disease, and high blood pressure; and cause blurred vision, sedation, palpitations, dizziness, constipation, and skin rashes. For colitis, doctors like to prescribe sulfasalazine (Azulfidine), which can pose serious health risks for people with kidney damage, liver damage, blood disorders, severe allergies, or bronchial asthma. One-third of the people who take this drug experience skin reactions, headaches, loss of appetite, vomiting, and an "apparently reversible" reduction in sperm count.

Dosage Options:

One dropper of concentrated extract or tincture (not the essential oil) daily, 1 tablespoon of fresh peppermint leaves in a cup of hot water three or four times a day, 1 to 2 teaspoons of dried leaves in a cup of water up to three times a day, or one or two enteric-coated peppermint oil pills standardized to contain 0.2 milliliter of the essential oil three times a day. Make sure you get coated capsules; the covering allows the herbal medicine to survive stomach acids and reach the intestines, where it can relax smooth muscles. For help against headaches, dilute some peppermint oil with a little alcohol and massage it into the temples.

Safety Rating: 3

Precautions:

Peppermint tea is virtually innocuous, but stronger forms of the herb could pose problems for some people. Those with achlorhydria (lack of a certain stomach acid) or liver disease should not take peppermint. Some especially cautious commentators say that people with gallbladder disease shouldn't take it either, even though the herb has proved helpful against the condition. Infants and small children should not ingest peppermint or even inhale the herb's vapors.

Do not ingest pure peppermint oil, and do not apply it topically. It may irritate the skin or cause dermatitis. Excessive external application or inhalation also may cause flushing or headaches. Prolonged excessive consumption of peppermint leaves might damage the liver or intestines. Some people might suffer heartburn, diarrhea, or other intestinal reactions, especially if coated capsules dissolve too quickly in the stomach.

PERIWINKLE *(Vinca minor)*

What It Is:

To some people in France, it's the "violet of the sorcerers," a reference to the plant's flowers and to its traditional use to ward off evil spirits. To many others in Europe and elsewhere in the world, it's known as myrtle and is more practically useful (and probably more effective) as an ornamental ground cover. Originally from Europe, periwinkle—with its tiny blue or purple flowers and shiny, dark green leaves—grows wild throughout eastern North America.

Therapeutic Uses:
🌿 High blood pressure, senility, stroke.
🔲 Folk uses: Chest pain, debility, diarrhea, dizziness, dropsy, headache, hemorrhoids, inflammation, intestinal disease, menstrual pain, mucous membrane inflammation, neuroses, nosebleeds, sore throat, tonsillitis, toothache, vaginal problems, weakness, wounds.

Medicinal Properties:
Periwinkle is a blood-related medicine, with the seemingly contradictory abilities to stop bleeding, increase blood circulation in the brain, and lower hypertension. Vincamine, an extract of one of its alkaloids, is a pharmaceutical in Europe (brands include Cerebroxine, Equipur, and Oxicebral, among many others), prescribed for arterial and cerebral circulatory disorders. It is not available in the United States.

Dosage Options:
One-half to 1 teaspoon of a liquid extract or 2 to 4 grams of the powdered herb daily.

Safety Rating: 1

Precautions:
Don't take periwinkle if you're bothered by constipation or have hypotension. Taking too much can sharply reduce blood pressure. In some animal experiments, the plant lowered globulin levels and caused symptoms of other blood disorders.

PHYLLANTHUS (*Phyllanthus*, various species)

What It Is:
In the West Indies, some people call the plant "seed on the leaf," a reference to the scattered arrangement of its small round fruit under the branches. This bitter, light green weed may grow up to 2 feet tall. Several *Phyllanthus* species exist, including *P. amarus, P. debilis,* and *P. fraternus.* They are difficult to tell apart and are often substituted for one another.

Therapeutic Uses:
🌿🌿 Hepatitis, jaundice.
🌿 Bacterial infections, HIV.
🔲 Folk uses: Colic, diabetes, diarrhea, dropsy, dysentery, eye inflammation, gonorrhea, indigestion, sores, tissue swelling, ulcers, urinary tract infections, water retention.

Medicinal Properties:
Little research has been conducted on this herb. In test tube experiments, phyllanthus extracts have displayed some ability to protect liver cells and deter aspects of HIV, the virus that causes AIDS. Other experiments have shown that an extract can

kill certain bacteria. In one study involving people, the herb was helpful in 22 of 37 people with hepatitis B.

Dosage Options:
One-half to a little more than 1 teaspoon of a liquid extract daily, 900 to 2,700 milligrams of the powdered herb daily for 3 months, or enough of a standardized phyllanthus supplement to provide 10 milligrams of sesquiterpenes a day.

Safety Rating: 1

Precautions:
None reported.

PICRORRHIZA *(Picrorrhiza kurroa)*

What It Is:
In Latin, *rhiza* means "root." If you want a sweet root, seek out glycyrrhiza, better known as licorice. If you want a harsh-tasting root, use picrorrhiza. The name translates literally as "bitter root." Although the roots of this low-growing, hairy, Himalayan perennial do impart a disagreeable flavor, the plant is pleasant to look at, with white to bluish purple flowers, and it has helpful medicinal properties.

Therapeutic Uses:
🌿🌿 Asthma, infections, osteoarthritis, psoriasis, spondylitis (an inflammation of the vertebrae), viral infections, vitiligo.
🌿 Allergies, autoimmune disorders, hepatitis, infections, lack of appetite, leishmaniasis, mushroom poisoning, pain, rheumatoid arthritis.
▦ Folk uses: Constipation, diarrhea, dropsy, flu, indigestion, jaundice, lung disease, malaria, snakebite.

Medicinal Properties:
Both standardized supplements and the herb can curb asthma and counteract viral infections. Picrorrhiza has triggered organ growth in lab rats whose livers were partially removed, spared them from chemically induced liver damage, stimulated immune system activity, and cooled inflammation. An extract from the plant called Picroliv is widely praised as a strong hepatic protector in India. Some studies suggest that it's at least as potent as the silymarin in milk thistle. Other research concludes that the kutkin in picrorrhiza is comparable or superior to milk thistle's silybinin for treating poisoning from amanita mushrooms. (See "Milk Thistle" on page 149.) There is no comparable pharmaceutical treatment for amanita poisoning.

Dosage Options:
One-quarter to 1 teaspoon of picrorrhiza extract or ½ to 2 grams of dried root daily.

Safety Rating: 1

Precautions:
Some people may experience a skin rash, diarrhea, or intestinal gas. You also may find the plant intolerably bitter.

PINEAPPLE *(Ananas comosus)*

What It Is:
When Christopher Columbus first encountered the pineapple in Guadeloupe in the early 1490s, he dubbed it "the pine of the Indies," an apt description for a fruit that looks like an overgrown green pinecone. *Piñas,* as they're called in many Spanish-speaking countries, soon found their way around the world, although they didn't reach Hawaii, now a major producer, until 1813. What we call the fruit is in fact a mass of flower heads that grow around one of the plant's stems. Each of those nubs on the peel is the dried-up remnant of a purple flower. In Central America, people sometimes cook and eat the long, tender, swordlike leaf shoots, although most of us prefer what's inside that knobby flower complex. The medicinal interest comes mostly from a proteolytic phytochemical called bromelain, which is present only in modest quantities or almost absent from the fruit.

Therapeutic Uses for Fruit:
🠾 Arthritis, blood clots, bruises, cancer, diarrhea, inflammation, lack of appetite, pain, sinus problems, sprains, strains, tissue swelling, ulcers, urinary tract infections, water retention, wounds.
▦ Folk uses: Constipation, gas, indigestion, kidney stones, labor, menstrual pain, neurasthenia, phlebitis, respiratory disease, thrombophlebitis, varicose veins, venereal disease, worms.

Therapeutic Uses for Bromelain:
🠾🠾 Arthritis, blood clots, bruises, indigestion, sinus problems, sprains, strains, tissue swelling, water retention.
🠾 Cancer, diarrhea, pain, ulcers, wounds.
▦ Folk uses: Menstrual pain, thrombophlebitis, varicose veins.

Medicinal Properties for Fruit:
The fruit contains protein-dissolving enzymes, notably bromelain, and another phytochemical called alpha-hydroxy acid, which exfoliates the skin. Neither substance appears in any significant concentration in whole pineapple fruit, but as isolated supplemental extracts, both are big therapeutic business. Let's look at the capabilities of each.

Medicinal Properties for Bromelain:

Concentrated primarily in the inedible stems, this phytochemical is particularly popular among athletes for treating all sorts of physical aches and injuries. It's been applied to and prescribed for everything from sprains, strains, twists, and pulls to bumps, bruises, and even arthritis—virtually any condition in which joints, muscles, or other tissues become bruised or inflamed. Studies indicate that bromelain simultaneously inhibits one prostaglandin involved in inflammatory processes but triggers the release of another prostaglandin that tamps down inflammation.

The enzyme also is said to thin the blood and heal bruises, countering the body's tendency to block off blood vessels and retain fluid at any injured, inflamed site. In a study of boxers, bruises and black-and-blue marks cleared up within 4 days for almost 80 percent of the pugilists who took a daily bromelain supplement. By contrast, only 14 percent of the boxers who did not take bromelain healed as soon. Other research demonstrates that bromelain helps the body eliminate substances related to arthritis and helps heal bruised, leaky capillaries.

Although bromelain backers say that these results are valid, others are skeptical about what they consider popular mythology. The research results are equivocal and, to some herbal authorities, not entirely convincing. Some question also exists about bromelain's absorption from the gut.

The extracted enzyme probably is of some value, but it may be overhyped. Nature gave us many similar proteolytic enzymes, a number of them more highly concentrated in the edible parts of other plants. Ginger is an excellent example (see "Ginger" on page 110). The zingibain it contains possesses some interesting protein-dissolving properties that might challenge bromelain's. It certainly appears more abundantly in the edible part of the plant than does bromelain in pineapple. In other words, with ginger you derive more of a medicinal effect from eating the whole food—the best way to benefit from herbal medicine.

Medicinal Properties for Alpha-Hydroxy Acid:

Alpha-hydroxy acid may or may not deserve its reputation as a wrinkle remover, skin smoother, acne eraser, and wound healer. In laboratory tests, it has helped dissolve substances that hold together dead skin cells. It also has thickened the upper, living layer of the epidermis, allowing skin to hold water and smooth out fine lines. Pineapple isn't the only, or even the best, source of alpha-hydroxy acid. It is present in many fruits, including apples and grapes, as well as in red wine, sugar cane, and milk.

Dosage Options:

Eat as much pineapple as you'd like. You can also try rubbing the inner peel on damaged skin several times a day. Don't expect to benefit from bromelain's anti-inflammatory effects by eating the fruit, however. The phytochemical appears only in low levels in the pulp, and less than half of that survives the digestive process. (Most of the bromelain is found in the stem, which, unlike any other fruit, runs through the whole pineapple. That's why pineapple slices have a hole in the middle.) Supplemental dosage options for isolated bromelain range from 80 to 320 milligrams daily to 250 to 500 milligrams three times a day.

Safety Rating:
For the fruit, **3**; for bromelain, **1**.

Precautions:
Few people have to worry about any side effects from eating pineapple. Indulge to your heart's content. As for bromelain, proponents claim that as much as 2 grams of the extract has been administered in studies with no ill effects. However, some people might get diarrhea or have other gastrointestinal reactions. If you're taking a prescription blood thinner, be careful with bromelain, which works similarly; taking the extract and the pharmaceutical simultaneously may thin your blood too much. Talk to an herb-savvy doctor, and you may be able to reduce your dependence on the synthetic medication. Also be careful if you're taking certain prescription antibiotics, especially for infections such as pneumonia, staphylococcus, and bronchitis. Some investigations say that bromelain increases blood and urinary levels of penicillin and tetracyclines.

PINE BARK *(Landes,* various species)

See "Grape; Grape Seed" on page 120.

PLANTAIN *(Plantago major)*

What It Is:
There are more than 200 species in the plantain family, including the well-known laxative psyllium (see "Psyllium" on page 178). The clan does not, however, include the banana-like fruit called plantain *(Musa paradisiaca),* whose common name comes from the Spanish word *plátano,* which means "plane tree." Plantain the weed, with its wide oval leaves and shoots of whitish or brownish green flowers, is indigenous to Eurasia but grows just about anywhere. If you live in a temperate climate in North America, there's a good chance you have this all-purpose herb right in your backyard.

Therapeutic Uses:
❧ Arthritis, bloody urine, breast cancer, bronchitis, colds, colon cancer, cystitis, dandruff, hemorrhoids, high blood pressure, high cholesterol, high triglycerides, psoriasis, thrush, ulcers, yeast infections.
▦ Folk uses: Diarrhea, dysentery.

Medicinal Properties:

Plantain has a long history of use as a treatment for a variety of skin woes, from dandruff and eczema to bug bites and minor cuts. The plant's juice is, in fact, antibacterial and quite soothing when applied to a burn. Like comfrey, it contains allantoin, an anti-inflammatory phytochemical that speeds wound healing, stimulates the growth of new skin cells, and gives the immune system a lift. Some European research has validated plantain's use in relieving bronchitis, sore throat, and respiratory complaints stemming from a cold.

Dosage Options:

One-half to 1 teaspoon of a liquid extract or tincture three times a day or 1 to 2 teaspoons of dried seeds in a glass of water daily. You can rub some of the fresh herb on bug bites and minor skin irritations.

Safety Rating: 2

Precautions:

Taking extremely large dosages might induce diarrhea or lower blood pressure. Some sensitive people might experience a skin rash or another allergic reaction. If you are allergic to psyllium, you may be allergic to plantain.

PLEURISY ROOT *(Asclepias tuberosa)*

What It Is:

Indigenous to Canada and the United States, this perennial herb's bright orange flowers, which bloom in the middle of summer, are a big attraction to butterflies, giving rise to another of its common names, butterfly weed. The more medicinally oriented name stems from its use among Native Americans to relieve serious respiratory problems, including pneumonia and the nasty lung inflammation known as pleurisy. Unlike other members of the milkweed family, the plant doesn't bleed a milklike sap. It does, however, grow pods filled with silk-tailed seeds.

Therapeutic Uses:

▓ Folk uses: Arthritis, asthma, bronchitis, bruises, colds, congestion, coughing, fever, flu, indigestion, lung disease, nasal problems, pain, pleurisy, pneumonia, stomachache, swelling, uterine disease.

Medicinal Properties:

Despite its name, pleurisy root's traditional medical applications have not been validated. Interestingly, the little research that has been conducted suggests a possible use in cardiac care. An extract of pleurisy root's asclepin strengthens heart contractions, perhaps better and more safely than the drug digoxin (Lanoxin).

Dosage Options:
One-half to 1 teaspoon of a root extract three times a day, ¼ to 1 teaspoon of a root tincture three times a day, or 1 tablespoon of the powdered root in a glass of a warm liquid daily.

Safety Rating: 1

Precautions:
Think long and hard before deciding to take this herb, perhaps doing so only on the advice of an herb-savvy physician. Large doses could upset your stomach or make you vomit. Some people might experience a skin reaction. Even low dosages of the extract may cause uterine contractions, so don't take the herb if you're pregnant or nursing. Pleurisy root also might interfere with heart medications, antidepressants, or prescription hormones. The plant itself is toxic to livestock, and intravenous extracts have been shown to be toxic to rabbits and rats.

PRICKLY ASH (*Zanthoxylum*, various species)

What It Is:
In the 1800s, prickly ash was often prescribed for toothaches, giving it the popular name toothache tree. In this regard, nineteenth-century practitioners took their cue from Native Americans, who used to chew on the bark to alleviate dental pain. Some 20 or 30 similar prickly ash species grow throughout the world, all of them unrelated to the plain old ash family. In the United States and Canada, two species predominate: northern prickly ash (*Z. americanum*) and southern prickly ash (*Z. clava-herculis*). Both are shrublike trees with sparsely thorned trunks and branches, delicately serrated leaves, white green flowers, and round red berries. It's not easy to tell the two apart. From Quebec south to Georgia and west to Oklahoma, you'll probably encounter northern prickly ash in woods and along rivers. From around Delaware south to Florida and west to Texas, southern prickly ash predominates. In the overlapping area, you'll find both.

Therapeutic Uses:
🌿 Dry mouth, high blood pressure, toothache.
▨ Folk uses: Arthritis, cancer, circulatory impairment, colds, coughing, cramps, dysentery, fever, heart disease, indigestion, inflammation, intermittent claudication, kidney disease, lung disease, neuroses, pancreatic problems, Raynaud's disease, sore throat, tonsillitis.

Medicinal Properties:
Too little medical research has been done on prickly ash to understand its therapeutic potential or confidently recommend its use. Some observers have said that it helps assuage toothache only by serving as a burning counterirritant. Others note

an analgesic aspect, pointing out that the plant's chelerythrine prolongs sleep induced by barbiturates. Does it really make a difference how the herb works when, in the end, it actually does ease a toothache? In animal studies, extracts blocked neuromuscular contractions and lowered blood pressure. Chewing on prickly ash bark makes your mouth water and gets your gastric juices flowing, which is probably why it's been prescribed in folk medicine for indigestion and stomach problems.

Dosage Options:
One-quarter to about ½ teaspoon of a liquid bark extract three times a day, ⅛ to ¼ teaspoon of a liquid berry extract daily, or ½ to 1 teaspoon of a bark tincture three times a day.

Safety Rating: 1

Precautions:
Because of its folkloric use as a uterine stimulant, you probably should not take prickly ash if you're pregnant or nursing. Its anticoagulant ability could compound the effects of any blood-thinning medications you take. Ingesting prickly ash has proved fatal to cattle, chicken, and fish, but not people.

PSYLLIUM *(Plantago ovata)*

What It Is:
To the experts and the herbalists, it's psyllium. To you, it's Metamucil, Fiberall, or many of the other brand-name laxatives. Seeds and seed cases from psyllium, an annual herb whose several varieties are native to the Mediterranean and western Asia, are the active ingredients in many commercial laxatives. The name is derived from *psylla,* the Greek word for "flea," a reference to the minuscule seeds.

Therapeutic Uses:
🍂🍂 Colitis, constipation, diarrhea, high cholesterol.
🍂 Coughing, cramps, diabetes, diverticulitis, dysentery, hemorrhoids, hepatitis, high blood pressure, high triglycerides, intestinal disease, irritable bowel syndrome, obesity, pregnancy, rectal problems, yeast infections.
▦ Folk uses: Boils, cystitis, dermatitis, gout, hardening of the arteries, hepatitis, lymph gland problems, psoriasis, stress, ulcers, urinary tract infections.

Medicinal Properties:
Credit the ingenuity of nature for devising a substance able to treat both diarrhea and constipation, depending on what ails you. Psyllium is indeed superior at alleviating these two contradictory complaints and several other bowel problems. The seeds' mucilage sucks up fluids, adding bulk to the stool and inhibiting diarrhea. To fight constipation, the seeds' absorption of liquids softens the stool, and the larger

volume helps provoke the intestinal contractions responsible for bowel movements. The easier action also comes in handy if you have hemorrhoids, inflammatory bowel disease, or diverticulitis. In one clinical study of people with hemorrhoids, 84 percent of the participants who took psyllium said they experienced less pain, less bleeding, and less itching upon going to the bathroom. Other research has demonstrated that mucilage, as a soluble fiber, helps lower cholesterol (and, to a lesser extent, triglycerides). It also may reduce high blood pressure.

Prescription Counterparts:
Unless you have a desire to pay higher prices and ingest sugar and artificial flavorings, give natural psyllium a try before turning to a brand-name product. For a better taste, mix it with your favorite juice.

Dosage Options:
One to 2 tablespoons of dried psyllium seeds or husks in a glass of water or juice daily, 2 teaspoons of fresh seeds or 1 teaspoon of fresh husks in a glass of water or juice one or more times a day, or ½ to 1 teaspoon of a liquid seed extract daily. Another option is 1,695 to 2,260 milligrams of powdered psyllium supplements three times a day. Once you take psyllium, drink more water and other liquids (see "Precautions").

Safety Rating: 3

Precautions:
Virtually none, as long as you drink a lot of water and other fluids. If you don't, you'll become constipated, perhaps seriously so. Don't take psyllium simultaneously with any other drug, no matter what it is. Separate the two by at least an hour. Otherwise, psyllium could lower your absorption of the medication and reduce its effectiveness. People with diabetes who give themselves insulin injections may have to keep a closer eye on their blood sugar levels; the mucilage may require a downward adjustment in your dosage. Don't take psyllium at all if you're taking loperamide (Imodium) or another drug designed to slow intestinal motility. A few sensitive people might suffer an allergic reaction to ingesting psyllium or inhaling the powdered seeds.

PUMPKIN *(Cucurbita pepo)*

What It Is:
This big orange gourd is a happy harbinger of fall. Pumpkin is indigenous to tropical areas of the Americas, where there is no temperate spring and fall, but it now grows almost anywhere. The next time you carve a pumpkin, be sure to save the seeds.

Therapeutic Uses:

🔹🔹 Bladder disease and stones.

🔹 Adenoma, cystitis, prostate enlargement (benign), prostatitis, roundworm, tapeworm.

▦ Folk uses: Bed-wetting, kidney inflammation, urinary pain.

Medicinal Properties:
In parts of Europe, handfuls of pumpkin seeds are standard treatment for benign prostate enlargement. The oil in pumpkin seeds is a provocative diuretic, but that doesn't fully explain their therapeutic effect on the prostate. The seeds also contain a strong concentration of phytochemicals called cucurbitacins, which in some studies have been shown to prevent a key chemical reaction in the condition—the transformation of testosterone into dihydrotestosterone. The delta-7-sterols may function even better for this. (For more information on the process, see "Saw Palmetto" on page 195.) Pumpkin seeds are rich in zinc and selenium, minerals that have been found to lower the risk of prostate cancer. The seeds also contain decent amounts of three gland-shrinking amino acids: alanine, glycine, and glutamic acid.

Dosage Options:
As many handfuls of dried pumpkin seeds as you'd like to eat.

Safety Rating: 3

Precautions:
None reported. Some researchers warn that some pumpkin seeds contain no cucurbitacins at all. Unfortunately, there's no way of knowing for sure without chemically analyzing every batch.

PYCNOGENOL

See "Grape; Grape Seed" on page 120.

PYGEUM *(Prunus africana)*

What It Is:
Some call this tree African cherry because it grows mostly in central Africa and on the off-coast island of Madagascar and is closely related to the cherry tree. Like the cherry, it's a member of the rose family. Pygeum sports small cherrylike berries, but they're very bitter. That's okay, though, because the fruit of this tree isn't what you're after. For health purposes, you want the bark. So many people want it, in fact, that

pygeum has become an endangered species in parts of Africa. When you rip off too much bark, you kill the tree. Fortunately, thanks to the Agroforestry Center in Nigeria, farmers in several African nations are being taught how to grow pygeum as a "living fence post tree," harvesting the bark judiciously and renewably, rather than rashly and destructively.

Therapeutic Uses:
 Bed-wetting, prostate enlargement (benign), urinary pain.
▦ Folk use: Urinary frequency.

Medicinal Properties:
If you're an older male at risk for prostate enlargement, benign or otherwise, this herb is helpful. When German researchers tested it on some 250 men with benign prostate enlargement, more than half noticed a benefit. Don't be duped by comparative studies between pygeum and saw palmetto (see "Saw Palmetto" on page 195). The two aren't competitors; they're teammates.

Dosage Options:
One hundred to 200 milligrams of a standardized supplement daily.

Safety Rating: 3

Precautions:
None reported, although some extremely sensitive people might suffer intestinal upset. A prostate problem is not something you should treat on your own. See "Saw Palmetto" on page 195, then see a physician trained in herbal medicine.

R

RASPBERRY *(Rubus idaeus)*

What It Is:
The fruit is so tasty—plucked right from the plant, in jellies and preserves, and as a juice, tea, vinegar, wine, or brandy—that it's easy to overlook the rest of the plant, a perennial or biennial shrub native to Europe and naturalized in North America. Native Americans made a tea from the root bark to ease inflamed eyes. Europeans

and other herbal advocates preferred to brew up the toothy leaves to treat diarrhea, colds, and stomach complaints, among other health problems.

Therapeutic Uses:
🍂 Colds, cramps, diarrhea, dysentery, flu, hemorrhoids, inflammation, intestinal disease, labor, menstrual pain, oral inflammation, sore throat, tonsillitis, uterine bleeding, wounds.

▦ Folk uses: Canker sores, coughing, diabetes, eye inflammation, fever, fever blisters, lung disease, morning sickness, nausea, prostatitis, skin problems, stomach disease, ulcers.

Medicinal Properties:
Despite the variety of folk applications, raspberry's most extensive use is to alleviate menstrual discomfort and facilitate childbirth. The little research conducted on the plant in these regards is contradictory. Some studies say that it can either relax or stimulate uterine muscles. Other experiments have found that it relaxes the uterus only during pregnancy. Still other studies show a uterine influence regardless of pregnancy. In pregnancy, the extract apparently normalizes uterine contractions and reduces their frequency. Scientists have isolated one substance in the extract that arouses smooth muscles, particularly those in the uterus, and another substance that quells uterine spasms.

Other phytochemicals in raspberry, notably the tannins, are astringent and help control some viruses and bacteria.

Dosage Options:
One to 2 teaspoons of crushed dried leaves in a cup of hot water up to six times a day, 384 to 1,152 milligrams of a standardized supplement three times a day, or 1 to 2 teaspoons of a liquid extract three times a day.

Safety Rating: 2

Precautions:
Any warning depends on which studies you believe. Some say the leaves should not be ingested in any form while you're pregnant and used during labor only under the supervision of a physician, if at all. Raspberry tea, however, is one of the most widely recommended herbal therapies for the entire course of pregnancy.

RED CLOVER (Trifolium pratense)

What It Is:
It rarely has four leaves (or leaflets, as botanists call them), but this species of clover nevertheless has always been a lucky charm against malevolence, whether mystical or medical. Red clover, so named for its pinkish or rose-colored flower heads, once

warded off witches and other evil forces, as well as a handful of more tangible threats, such as respiratory and skin problems. More modern herbal experts value the plant for its strong concentration of natural estrogens and its potential to thwart cancer. Red clover came from Europe but is naturalized across much of the United States, notably in Vermont, where it's the official state flower.

Therapeutic Uses:
🐛🐛 Menopause.

🐛 Bronchitis, cancer (especially breast; prevention and treatment), colds, congestion, coughing, cramps, lung disease.

▦ Folk uses: Asthma, dermatitis, eczema, indigestion, jaundice, menstrual pain, psoriasis, syphilis, tuberculosis, venereal disease, whooping cough.

Medicinal Properties:
Like kudzu, soy, and flaxseed (see "Kudzu" on page 136, "Soybean" on page 204, and "Flax" on page 104), red clover possesses a strong concentration of natural estrogens, plant world equivalents of human female hormones. Phytoestrogens perform functions in the body similar to those of natural and synthetic estrogens, relieving menopause- and menstruation-related problems and perhaps protecting against osteoporosis and cancer of the breast, colon, and prostate. When the body's own supply is low, the phytoestrogens step in and help pick up the slack. If you're taking prescription female hormones, which have been linked to breast cancer, the milder phytoestrogens again step in and prevent the synthetics from interacting with tissue cells. Soy is perhaps the best known and studied source of phytoestrogens, but that doesn't mean it's necessarily the best source.

In one study of postmenopausal women, those who abided by a diet high in red clover, soy, and flaxseed for 2 weeks all had higher levels of the female hormone. Levels dropped when the women stopped the phytoestrogen-rich diet. In a very small 2-week animal study of three heifers fed a large quantity of red clover, researchers documented measurable size increases in teats and certain uterine proportions. Scientists have identified at least four phytoestrogenic isoflavones in red clover—biochanin-A, daidzein, genistein, and formononetin. Unlike soy, many clover species contain all four of these substances.

Genistein, the most publicized of the phytoestrogens, seems to be associated not only with fewer female-specific complaints but a lower incidence of several hormone-dependent cancers. Genistein inhibits a process called angiogenesis, through which tumor cells encourage the creation of new blood vessels. Biochanin-A also deters some carcinogenic actions, at least in petri dish experiments.

No clinical studies have documented an anticancer benefit of red clover, but it deserves the same scientific consideration as soy. The herb's natural balance of phytochemicals perhaps explains its inclusion in the Hoxsey formula, a controversial alternative cancer treatment that also includes, among other herbs, licorice, prickly ash, buckthorn, and cascara sagrada.

Prescription Counterparts:
Along with kudzu and soy, red clover's balance of natural phytoestrogens may be a better first choice for menopause- and PMS-related problems than strong, out-of-balance synthetic drugs. As for cancer prevention and treatment, the issue remains hotly debated. The evidence suggests that any phytoestrogen (not just genistein) will help prevent hormone-dependent tumors, although naysayers argue that the compounds, like their synthetic rivals, also stimulate the spread of malignant breast (and presumably prostate) cells. And for all the hubbub over Hoxsey, it's probably safer than some of the devastating chemotherapies out there.

Dosage Options:
One to 3 teaspoons of dried flowers in a cup of hot water three times a day, 1,050 milligrams of a standardized supplement, ¼ to ½ teaspoon of a liquid extract, or ¼ to 1 teaspoon of a tincture. Or drink a tea made with 1 to 2 tablespoons of fresh flowers up to three times a day.

Safety Rating: 3

Precautions:
Red clover is safe in amounts that people normally would consume, but consult a physician before taking it if you're pregnant or nursing an infant. Pregnant animals have had miscarriages after grazing heavily on clover. Some research has linked a meat-free diet high in plant estrogens to certain birth defects in male babies. Other studies suggest that the phytoestrogens, especially formononetin, could cause growth disorders, infertility, hives, or skin rashes. Among cattle, ingesting fermented red clover has caused diarrhea and dermatitis and reduced milk production. (But we're talking about huge quantities of clover here, not a couple of capsules a day.)

REHMANNIA; CHINESE FOXGLOVE (*Rehmannia glutinosa*)

What It Is:
Most of this plant's leaves grow at ground level, with a few smaller, egg-shaped, short-stalked leaves up the stem beneath purple-veined, yellow to purplish brown flowers. Sounds like foxglove, doesn't it? But rehmannia is only a foot or so tall, and the 10 or so species are all from eastern Asia, with this plant native to and widely grown in China (hence its common name). It's occasionally cultivated as an ornamental in the United States.

Therapeutic Uses:
🌿🌿 Arthritis, asthma, high blood pressure, hives, kidney disease.
🌿 Anemia, autoimmune disorders, dermatitis, eczema, hepatitis, hyperthyroidism (Graves' disease), thrombosis, urinary bleeding.

⊞ Folk uses: Backache, cataracts, constipation, coughing, diabetes, dizziness, fever, graying hair, hemorrhage, insomnia, lumbago, measles, menstrual pain and irregularities, nosebleeds, palpitations, rashes, restlessness, semen discharge (involuntary and without orgasm), sore throat, tinnitus, tongue inflammation, weakness.

Medicinal Properties:
Some researchers have reported good clinical success with a rehmannia extract used against arthritis pain and asthma. Other studies show that rehmannia encourages fluid excretion, relaxes blood vessels, and stimulates the adrenal glands.

Dosage Options:
One teaspoon to 1 tablespoon of a liquid extract daily or 5 grams of ground root in a cup of hot water up to three times a day. Or steep about ½ ounce of ground root in a pint of red wine and drink a glass every day.

Safety Rating: 1

Precautions:
Some people may get dizzy, feel lethargic, or experience heart palpitations after ingesting rehmannia. The root, whether raw or cooked, could cause diarrhea. The raw root also may cause loss of appetite or upset stomach.

RHUBARB *(Rheum palmatum)*

What It Is:
Don't you dare make a pie with this species of rhubarb. If you do, you won't find it very filling for very long. Medicinal rhubarb, as it's known, is a strong laxative. In China, where it is native, the plant is called *da huang,* or "great yellow," a reference to its yellow rhizome, which Asian herbalists have ground up into a purgative powder for the past 5,000 years. By contrast, edible rhubarb *(R. rhabarbarum* or *R. x hybridum)* has been cultivated in Europe since the 1700s. Its root, too, was tried as an herbal laxative, but, except perhaps in large quantities, it's not very effective. Quite the contrary, the root is poisonous, as are the leaves in large quantities. The stalks are the edible parts of the plant.

Therapeutic Uses:
❧❧ Constipation, dysentery, endometriosis, hepatitis, high blood pressure, high cholesterol, high triglycerides, intestinal inflammation.
❧ Aggression, cancer, diarrhea, flu, gallbladder problems, gas, gingivitis, hemorrhage, hemorrhoids, herpes, intestinal pain, irritability, jaundice, kidney disease, oral inflammation, pancreatitis, preeclampsia (pregnancy-related high blood pressure), sores, ulcers, vaginal inflammation.

⧆ Folk uses: Appendicitis, burns, carbuncles, delirium, eye inflammation, fever, gastric bleeding, headache, indigestion, intestinal pain, lack of menstruation, low blood pressure, nosebleeds, obesity, pain, pregnancy, shingles, stomachache, swelling, tongue inflammation, toothache, vomiting of blood, wounds.

Medicinal Properties:

The various phytochemicals in medicinal rhubarb exert opposing therapeutic effects in different dosages. In very small amounts, the astringent tannins help inhibit diarrhea; in larger amounts, the anthraquinones react with bacteria in the digestive tract to create compounds that trigger intestinal contractions for a bowel movement. (The high fiber content of medicinal rhubarb helps somewhat, too.) Some herbal experts say that the phytochemical combination comes in especially handy for relieving constipation if you have hemorrhoids (because of the astringent action of the tannins). Chinese researchers have also found some help against ulcers. In one study of about 300 people with ulcers, 90 percent of the *da huang* users said they felt better within just a few days.

Dosage Options:

Up to 1 teaspoon of the powdered root as a tea one or two times a day, up to 1 tablespoon of a tincture daily, or ½ to 2 teaspoons of a liquid extract daily. A standardized supplement gives more for reliable results.

Safety Rating: 1

Precautions:

As with any laxative, natural or synthetic, don't take medicinal rhubarb for more than several days, and discontinue it if you get diarrhea. Regular use could be habit-forming (your body could come to depend on it for a bowel movement). Don't use medicinal rhubarb if you're pregnant or nursing, as the anthraquinones can leach into breast milk. Some experts caution that you shouldn't use the herb if you have arthritis, hemorrhoids, kidney disease, an intestinal obstruction, irritable bowel syndrome, colitis, or Crohn's disease. Other researchers claim that the use of anthraquinone laxatives triples the incidence of colon cancer.

ROSE HIPS *(Rosa canina)*

What It Is:

Pick up a bottle of vitamin C, read the label, and you're quite likely to find the ascorbic acid accompanied by rose hips. Rose hips are actually fruit, and they sort of resemble small, oval or spherical cherries. They form near the top of five-petaled flowers that vary in color from whitish to deep pink. The plant from which this particular fruit comes isn't your common garden rose (although all roses have hips) but the wild dog rose, whose leaves are greener and smoother than the more familiar ornamentals. This plant does have thorny stems, however, which may have given rise to its original common name, dag (or dagger) rose.

Therapeutic Uses:
- Capillary fragility.
- Folk uses: Arthritis, chills, colds, dropsy, flu, gastritis, gout, headache, infections, sciatica, sores, sore throat, stomach disease, stress, thirst, urinary pain.

Medicinal Properties:
Rose hips' therapeutic value comes, in part, from their vitamin C content, although they're not very exceptional sources of this antioxidant. A few other mild phytochemicals help out, too.

Dosage Options:
One-quarter to ½ cup of fresh rose hips daily, up to 3 teaspoons of fresh hips in a cup of hot water up to three times a day, or 1 to 2 grams or more of dried hips in a cup of hot water daily.

Safety Rating: 3

Precautions:
None reported.

ROSEMARY *(Rosmarinus officinalis)*

What It Is:
This shrubby herb, with pale blue (occasionally white or pink) flowers and gray green, pinelike (and piney-smelling) foliage, provides a familiar fragrance in both the bathroom and the kitchen. Its essential oil is used to scent toiletries; its dried leaves are a flavorful addition to stews, soups, and meats. In ancient Greece, the aroma of this spice, native to the Mediterranean from Portugal and Spain south to Morocco and Tunisia, scented the halls of academe: Students wore sprigs on their heads while they studied to enhance their memory. (They may have been keeping their hair healthy and staving off baldness, too, as later herbalists would claim of the plant.) Shakespeare, too, made reference to the mnemonic medicine, which gave rise to the plant's title, "herb of remembrance." Keep that in mind as you read about the other disease-fighting assets of this mint-family member.

Therapeutic Uses:
- Arthritis, circulatory problems, gallbladder problems, indigestion, lack of appetite, liver disease, sciatica.
- Alzheimer's disease, cataracts, bruises, cancer (especially breast), diabetes, drowsiness, gas, gastric disease, hardening of the arteries, heart disease, intestinal

disease, lethargy, low blood pressure, migraine, muscle pain, nerve pain, paralysis, rib pain (pleurodynia), septic shock, sprains, stomachache, varicose veins.

☒ Folk uses: Eczema, hair loss, headache, wounds.

Medicinal Properties:

Rosemary gives us much to remember—and the phytochemical "string around the finger" through which to do so. Some six or so substances in the herb (several of which are readily absorbed through the skin) help prevent the breakdown of the brain chemical acetylcholine, a deficiency of which has been implicated in Alzheimer's disease. It contains good concentrations of two dozen or so antioxidants. (Oxidation also figures in the brain deterioration process.) Other compounds trigger better blood circulation throughout the body, including the brain. The antioxidants also help protect the capillaries and ward off hardening of the arteries and heart disease. In this regard, rosemary's diosmin might be even better than the rutin in horse chestnut (see "Horse Chestnut" on page 127), pansies, and violets. Your eyes also benefit from antioxidants, as well as from at least four recognized anticataract chemicals. The essential oil's cineole arouses the central nervous system and serves as a natural pick-me-up. In laboratory experiments, the oil also has been shown to lower blood sugar. All these documented actions are cutting-edge phytomedicine, but many of rosemary's traditional uses also are backed up by science, including encouraging better release of digestive acids and dispelling intestinal gas.

Prescription Counterparts:

No synthetic pharmaceutical exists for generating better blood flow to the brain. The primary anti-Alzheimer's drug, tacrine (Cognex), causes vomiting, nausea, an increased likelihood of liver problems (including jaundice), and a greater risk of ulcers. Rosemary (and the similarly acting sage) is a perfect complementary adjunct to *Ginkgo biloba* in your herbal arsenal against Alzheimer's disease and the loss of cerebral blood circulation (see "Sage" on page 190 and "Ginkgo" on page 112).

Dosage Options:

One-half to 1 teaspoon of a liquid shoot extract three times a day or 1 teaspoon of chopped fresh or dried rosemary leaves steeped in a cup of hot water every day.

Safety Rating: 3

Precautions:

None reported with wise use of the whole herb. If you ingest a lot, your urine might take on a reddish tinge. A rosemary-induced discoloration is not a sign of a problem, but reddish, bloody urine is a warning that something is wrong. If you're taking rosemary and see the symptom, don't panic, but do consult a doctor just to make sure. The essential oil is toxic, so you shouldn't ingest it undiluted. If you do, you might suffer some irritation of the stomach, intestines, or kidneys. You also may notice a skin reaction. People with epilepsy should be careful, because rosemary contains camphor, a volatile oil known for causing convulsions.

RUE *(Ruta graveolens)*

What It Is:
A pretty perennial with tiny, daisylike, yellow flowers, rue may seem innocuous, but it's actually somewhat toxic. The ancient Romans did rely on the herb, which is native to Europe but naturalized in parts of the United States, to cure a variety of ailments, however. In the sixteenth to eighteenth centuries, its distinctive smell led to its reputation for repelling fleas, lice, and other vermin (in the Amazon, it repels bad luck), as well as for overcoming poisoning by everything from snakebite to noxious mushrooms.

Therapeutic Uses:
✒ Coughing, cramps, indigestion, insect infestations, intestinal disease, menstrual pain, worms.
▨ Folk uses: Diarrhea, earache, fever, infections, liver disease, oral inflammation, skin problems, toothache, uterine disease.

Medicinal Properties:
Rue's essential oil apparently is repugnant to vermin, and compounds do indeed calm muscle spasms and ease coughing. The plant also served as the first source of the capillary-protecting phytochemical rutin. But the trade-off may be too dear. Rue can, in large doses, provoke abortion-strength uterine contractions and other harmful side effects (see "Precautions"). We now have far better and safer sources of rutin, including buckwheat (see "Buckwheat" on page 54), eucalyptus, horse chestnut, mulberry leaves, pansies, and violets.

Dosage Options:
Do not ingest this herb, even though it's readily available at health food stores. Don't be tempted by dosage recommendations on various products (see "Precautions").

Safety Rating:
Do not take.

Precautions:
You may rue the day that you ingest rue. It's a poisonous plant, whether ingested or applied topically. Yes, it's loaded with spasm-calming natural compounds, but it may cause miscarriage, intestinal pain, vomiting, convulsions, limb twitching, and perhaps even death. Just touching it can cause a skin reaction in some people, and external use can result in serious dermatitis when you're out in the sun.

SAGE *(Salvia officinalis)*

What It Is:
This evergreen, mint-family perennial is native to the Balkans and the Mediterranean region. Its bluish purple flowers and grayish green leaves have been a culinary and medicinal staple for some 2,000 years. In the 1600s, it was reputed to confer immortality. That claim likely is overblown, but sage probably can make your life, however long it might be, a little healthier.

Therapeutic Uses:
🌿🌿 Indigestion, lack of appetite, oral inflammation, perspiration (especially if excessive), rhinitis, sore throat.

🌿 Alzheimer's disease, arthritis, cancer, fever, gingivitis, gum bleeding, hoarseness, inflammation, intestinal inflammation, sores, stomach disease, tongue inflammation, tonsillitis.

▨ Folk uses: Acne, bug bites, canker sores, coughing, cramps, depression, dermatitis, diarrhea, excessive breast milk, hot flashes, infertility, laryngitis, menstrual pain, mucous membrane inflammation, night sweats, sprains, tuberculosis, wounds.

Medicinal Properties:
If you're going to Scarborough Fair, you're going on more than a musical odyssey. Whether they knew it or not, Simon and Garfunkel revealed a lot of phytochemical common sense in their famous song. Like parsley (see "Parsley" on page 164), sage helps freshen your breath, and like rosemary (see "Rosemary" on page 187) and thyme, the antioxidant-rich sage helps maintain the brain's concentration of the neurochemical acetylcholine. Europeans also used to rub the somewhat gritty leaves on their teeth and gums to sand off plaque. The plant's tannins are astringent and antiseptic, a big help in preventing gingivitis. Six or so other chemicals assist by fighting inflammation in the body. Some observers say that sage might be as effective as the sanguinarine (see "Bloodroot" on page 45) that's found in some toothpastes. All of these qualities come in handy for treating laryngitis, tonsillitis, and other oral inflammation.

Prescription Counterparts:
Sage possesses much the same anti-Alzheimer's potential as rosemary and could work well in combination with *Ginkgo biloba* (see "Ginkgo" on page 112) in fighting

off the disease. Orthodox medicine's main synthetic weapon against Alzheimer's is tacrine (Cognex), which raises the risk for ulcers and for jaundice and other liver problems. The drug also tends to make you vomit.

Dosage Options:
One-quarter to 1 teaspoon of a liquid leaf extract three times a day, 2 to 4 tablespoons of fresh leaves daily, or 2 teaspoons of the dried herb in a cup of hot water daily. You can drink the tea or just gargle with it.

Safety Rating: 3

Precautions:
Consuming sage leaves poses no problem for most people. Supplemental extracts and maybe even the tea, however, might be problematic if used to excess or for a prolonged period. The reason is the presence of the phytochemical thujone, which could cause convulsions, dizziness, hot flashes, or a rapid heartbeat.

ST. JOHN'S WORT *(Hypericum perforatum)*

What It Is:
Perky, star-shaped, yellow flowers burst forth from this plant around June 24, St. John's Day in the Christian calendar. If you pinch the leaves or the petals, out oozes a reddish purple stain—the "blood" of St. John. St. John's wort originated in Europe but now grows wild in Africa, Asia, Australia, North America, and South America. You'll find it throughout the United States, perhaps under the name Klamath weed on the West Coast. In California, it's classified as a wild weed that some people think should be eradicated. The USDA has even erected a monument to itself for checking the rampant growth of what arguably is one of the finest depression-fighting medicines humanity has ever seen (or synthesized).

Therapeutic Uses:
🌿🌿 Anxiety, burns, depression, dermatitis, indigestion, myalgia, seasonal affective disorder (SAD), wounds.
🌿 Alcoholism, arthritis, chickenpox, cold sores, congestion, cytomegalovirus, ear inflammation, flu, gastroduodenitis (inflammation of the stomach and duodenum), hemorrhage, hepatitis (including viral hepatitis), herpes, HIV, insomnia, menopause, nervousness, nerve pain, neuroses, pain, sciatica, stress, sunburn, vitiligo.
▦ Folk uses: Bed-wetting, bruises, colds, coughing, cramps, cuts, diarrhea, dysentery, excessive menstrual bleeding, gallbladder problems, hemorrhoids, hysteria, jaundice, kidney disease, lack of appetite, menstrual pain, parasitic infections, radiation exposure, respiratory disease, sores, ulcers, worms.

Medicinal Properties:

Thanks to phytochemicals such as hyperforin and hypericin, St. John's wort helps brighten the moods of people with mild to moderate depression and anxiety. It also helps get people out of the winter doldrums, a syndrome called seasonal affective disorder (SAD), although it is less effective against the up-and-down mood swings of bipolar depression.

St. John's wort works not only as well as some prescription medications but much like them, too, only more comprehensively and safely. Like selective serotonin reuptake inhibitors (SSRIs) such as fluoxetine hydrochloride (Prozac) and sertraline hydrochloride (Zoloft), it maintains brain levels of the mood-regulating chemical serotonin. And in much the same fashion as monoamine oxidase inhibitors (MAOIs) such as phenelzine sulfate (Nardil) and tranylcypromine sulfate (Parnate), it increases the concentrations of two other brain chemicals, dopamine and norepinephrine. As a bonus, it also increases melatonin and, perhaps, gamma-aminobutyric acid (GABA) levels. For 80 percent of more than 3,000 people participating in German research, taking St. John's wort extracts completely or partially reversed their depressive states.

Wounds of all kinds heal more rapidly and with less scarring under the influence of St. John's wort oils and ointments. Antibiotic, anti-inflammatory, and analgesic compounds help against cuts, scrapes, punctures, and burns from heat, electrical shocks, and even radiation. These compounds would, on their own, help ease herpes-related sores, but St. John's wort adds antiviral might. In the laboratory, that virus-fighting power has shown some potential against HIV.

Prescription Counterparts:

Of the more than two dozen strictly conducted clinical studies of St. John's wort, several have evaluated the herb's efficacy in comparison with standard antidepressant drugs, and the natural medicine has consistently proved itself superior or equal to its synthetic rivals. Not that it necessarily lifts low spirits to measurably higher levels than the pharmaceuticals, but it certainly can work about as well, and it imposes few or none of the drugs' unwanted consequences, which can include nausea, sexual dysfunction, headache, diarrhea, dry mouth, and insomnia, to name just a few. St. John's wort is far less expensive, too.

Dosage Options:

For a consistent therapeutic effect against mild depression or SAD, a standardized supplement containing 0.3 percent hypericin per capsule (in better brands, that translates to about 300 milligrams of a certified-potency extract) three times a day. Ingest at least 1 milligram of hypericin daily. Some supplements may be standardized for 3 percent hyperforin instead of 0.3 percent hypericin.

For herpes cold sores, steep 1 to 2 teaspoons of the dried herb in a cup of hot water. Drink the tea and apply it topically once or twice a day for up to 6 weeks. For cuts, scrapes, and burns, consider applying St. John's wort oil topically. You can make your own by steeping several teaspoons of the fresh herb in a carrier oil, such as evening primrose. For immune enhancement, take ½ to 1 teaspoon of a tincture or liquid extract three times a day.

Some potato chips and snack foods are flavored with a little St. John's wort. Note the qualifying "a little." Despite any therapeutic claims that might be made on the packages, these foods probably do not contain enough of the herb to make a difference in your disposition. If they do contain at least a tincture-level amount at a competitive price, they might be worth your while. Read the labels.

Safety Rating: 2

Precautions:

Few people have anything to be concerned about. If you have fair skin, you might become more sensitive to the sun, a curious possibility in that topically applied St. John's wort oil guards against sunburn and hastens wound healing. With a little sunscreen and a watchful eye to the amount of time you spend outdoors, you should be fine. Be careful, too, if you're taking prescription antidepressants. Given its verified effectiveness, St. John's wort certainly could alter the physiologic impact of MAOIs and SSRIs. Instead of shying away from the herb, as some overly cautious herbalists advise, talk to your physician. By using St. John's wort, perhaps you can get by with smaller doses of the pharmaceutical or end your reliance entirely.

In February 2000, the FDA issued a warning that St. John's wort, by triggering a particular enzyme in the body, could weaken the effectiveness of certain HIV medications—specifically, indinavir (Crixivan)—as well as certain antirejection drugs prescribed for heart transplant patients. If this is true, the FDA, in the name of completeness, should have added that grapefruit juice, by inhibiting the very same enzyme, may more than compensate for whatever action St. John's wort might effect.

SARSAPARILLA (*Smilax*, various species)

What It Is:

When the bowlegged cowpoke sauntered through the saloon's swinging doors, swaggered past his poker-playing pardners, bellied up to the bar, and ordered a "sasperilly," he may very well have wanted only to wet his whistle. More likely, though, he was seeking a cure for syphilis. Since European explorers arrived in America in the early sixteenth century, the root of this tropical vine, whose several thorny species belong to the lily family, was thought to be a cure for this sexually transmitted disease. In the mid-1800s, even the U.S. Pharmacopeia listed it as an official syphilis treatment, and sarsaparilla went on to be billed as a general blood-purifying, rejuvenative tonic for any number of complaints. One of the many species, *S. officinalis,* is still around in health food stores, promoted as a builder of muscle mass and reviver of the libido.

Therapeutic Uses:

❰ Arthritis, cancer, dermatitis, fever, gonorrhea, inflammation, intestinal disease, irritable bowel syndrome, psoriasis, stomach disease, urinary tract infections.

▣ Folk uses: Dysentery, eczema, erectile dysfunction, indigestion, kidney disease, leprosy, syphilis.

Medicinal Properties:

Sarsaparilla won't cure syphilis, nor will it do much of what its promoters claim it will do. In some clinical efforts, certain root phytochemicals, called saponins, have soothed psoriasis, most likely by disabling bacterial components called endotoxins that, in excess, can overtax the liver and aggravate inflammatory processes in the body. Endotoxins show up in the bloodstreams of people with psoriasis, arthritis, and gout. Saponins prevent endotoxins from being absorbed, thus lightening the load on the liver. That could explain sarsaparilla's blood-purifying reputation. As for the link to big muscles and a big libido? Nice try, but no cigar. True, at least one saponin, sarsapogenin, like diosgenin, can be converted into a sex steroid—but only by a chemist, not by your body.

Dosage Options:

Two 450-milligram capsules two or three times a day, 1½ teaspoons to 1 tablespoon of a liquid rhizome extract daily, ⅓ to 1 ounce of dried sarsaparilla root in 3 cups of hot water daily, 1 to 2 teaspoons of powdered root in a cup of hot water up to three times a day, ¼ to ½ teaspoon of sarsaparilla tincture up to three times a day, or 2 to 4 tablespoons of fresh roots daily.

Safety Rating: 3

Precautions:

Most people won't have any problems with sarsaparilla. Some people might get nauseous. Extremely large doses over a long period could harm the kidneys or the gastrointestinal tract. Think twice about taking sarsaparilla if you're also taking a pharmaceutical. The saponins magnify the effects of some drugs and reduce the effectiveness of others.

SASSAFRAS *(Sassafras albidum)*

What It Is:

Like sarsaparilla (see the previous entry), this once-popular plant has fallen out of favor. The aromatic, sweet-tasting sassafras was regarded as a blood-purifying, all-purpose tonic for whatever ails you, including syphilis. The pleasing flavor made it a favored tea on both sides of the Atlantic. For a while, only tobacco topped this eastern North American native as an export to Europe. Sassafras livened up the taste of chewing gum, toothpastes, and beverages (notably root beer) until the 1960s, when research established that one primary chemical in its volatile oil, safrole, causes cancer. The FDA then banned sassafras's use in food unless the safrole is removed.

Therapeutic Uses:

Fever.

Folk uses: Acne, arthritis, breast inflammation (mastitis), colds, dermatitis, eye inflammation, flu, gout, high blood pressure, intestinal disease, kidney disease, liver disease, measles, mucous membrane inflammation, pain, poison ivy, respiratory disease, stomachache, syphilis, urinary tract infections.

Medicinal Properties:

As Native Americans knew, sassafras encourages the excretion of urine and lowers body temperature. But its sweet taste and fever-reducing potential may come at a high cost. The tree's wood contains 1 to 2 percent of an oil that may be about 80 percent safrole, which, in its pure form, is a tumor-generating, gene-altering, hallucinogenic liver toxin. Even without the safrole, the tree's oil has caused tumors in lab animals. (No volatile oil, whether from sassafras or any other plant, should ever be ingested in pure form. See "Precautions.")

Dosage Options:

To be on the safe side, don't drink sassafras tea or take it supplementally.

Safety Rating: 1

Precautions:

Sassafras shouldn't be ingested or applied to the skin for any length of time, if at all. The question is how much of the pure oil's peril is imparted via judicious use of the herbal medicine. Ingesting as little as 1 teaspoon of the volatile oil has killed one adult, and just a few drops might be enough to kill a child. Some experts claim that just one cup of sassafras tea contains more than enough safrole to pose a high hazard. Other herbal experts dismiss the warning, saying that levels of safrole are less carcinogenic than the ethanol in a bottle of beer.

SAW PALMETTO (Serenoa repens)

What It Is:

To the Seminoles of what is now the southeastern United States, the reddish brown to black berries on this palm-family shrub were good food. How the Seminoles ate them, we'll never know, for the berries taste terrible and stink to high heaven. Only later were they used to ease upset stomachs and insomnia, among other complaints. None of the traditional uses heralded saw palmetto's current status as the premier treatment, natural or synthetic, for prostate problems.

Therapeutic Uses:

🌿🌿🌿 Prostate enlargement (benign).

🌿🌿 Gallbladder problems, hair loss, inflammation, prostatitis, urethral inflammation.

🌿 Cystitis, micromastia (abnormally small breasts).

▦ Folk uses: Asthma, bronchitis, colds, coughing, debility, dysentery, low libido, mucous membrane inflammation, migraine, stomachache, stomach disease, testicular problems, urinary excess, urinary pain or problems, uterine disease.

Medicinal Properties:

Saw palmetto frequently equals and sometimes exceeds pharmaceuticals for treating benign prostate hypertrophy (BPH), the noncancerous enlargement of the prostate that strikes at least half of all men 50 years old and as many as 90 percent of all men 70 years old and up. The condition makes urination difficult, perhaps painful, and leaves a man unable to empty his bladder thoroughly, resulting in frequent visits to the bathroom, especially at night. More than a dozen clinical studies involving almost 3,000 men have verified saw palmetto's ability to markedly alleviate BPH symptoms, increasing urinary flow and decreasing the number of sleep-disturbing jaunts to the john—without the libido-reducing side effects of its pharmaceutical rival (see "Prescription Counterparts"). The herb helps more men than the synthetic drug, and it gets the job done faster.

In yet another contrast to the doctor-preferred drug, saw palmetto's phytochemical cornucopia works on several levels. Like the pharmaceutical, it curbs an enzyme that converts testosterone into a hormonal form called dihydrotestosterone, which spurs prostate cells to reproduce. But it also prevents dihydrotestosterone from interacting with prostate cells and quenches tissue inflammation, neither of which the drug seems to do. Dihydrotestosterone also is the leading suspect behind male pattern baldness. Informal, anecdotal evidence indicates that saw palmetto stems hair loss and triggers regrowth, but so far no clinical studies have been conducted to validate or negate the claims. Nor has science tried to verify reports that berry extracts stimulate blood flow to the genitals, support the thyroid's regulation of sexual development, and increase both lactation and breast size.

Prescription Counterparts:

Chemists worked long, hard, and at high cost to make a medicine that combats BPH. The result was finasteride (Proscar), which does not work as well as saw palmetto, inflicts many more side effects, and costs about three times as much. Even the *Journal of the American Medical Association* concludes that the berry extract works as well and with fewer side effects. Here's how the drug and saw palmetto match up.

How many benefit? Finasteride relieves urinary symptoms for less than 50 percent of the BPH-affected men who take it. Saw palmetto works for more than 80 percent of its users.

What is the trade-off? Finasteride lowers libidinous urges and impairs erectile ability. Saw palmetto impairs erectile ability and tames the libido in only a comparatively few men.

When does it go to work? Men have to take finasteride for at least 6 months before it shows any benefit. Saw palmetto's benefits become apparent within 3 months.

How comprehensive is it? Finasteride inhibits only the creation of dihydrotestosterone. Saw palmetto not only deters the creation of dihydrotestosterone but also inhibits the hormone from interacting with the prostate.

How does it affect the gland? Finasteride significantly shrinks the size of the prostate. Saw palmetto has no appreciable impact on the gland's size.

How safe is it? According to advocates of the drug and the FDA, any woman who might conceive a child should not touch finasteride, even briefly. Saw palmetto, as far as we know, poses no such threat.

Dosage Options:
The preferred therapeutic dosage and form for an enlarged prostate is 640 milligrams daily of a standardized supplement containing 320 milligrams of a certified-potency fruit extract and 90 percent fatty acids and biologically active sterols. Better brands include similar wording on their labels. Other dosages include 1,200 to 1,800 milligrams of a nonstandardized supplement, a little more than ¼ teaspoon of a liquid fruit extract, about 1 teaspoon of a liquid whole-herb extract, or 2 to 3 teaspoons of fresh saw palmetto berries every day.

Safety Rating: 3

Precautions:
Because saw palmetto works much like finasteride, logic dictates that whatever warnings are applicable to the drug should apply to the herb as well. But according to comparative clinical studies, saw palmetto is remarkably free of such side effects and consequences. Only a few men taking the herb have complained about a decline in sexual function or libido. Some sensitive people might experience a little gastric upset. The research is contradictory on whether the herb affects levels of a marker called prostate-specific antigen (PSA), which is used to gauge the risk of later developing prostate cancer. Finasteride reduces PSA levels. Some studies say that saw palmetto does, too; other studies say that it does not. As for the red flag that women who want to bear a child shouldn't touch the pharmaceutical, no evidence comes close to indicating that they shouldn't touch saw palmetto berries.

SCHISANDRA (Schisandra chinensis)

What It Is:
The Chinese call this member of the magnolia vine family *wu-wei-zi*, which translates as "five-flavor seeds." When you munch on the berries, they simultaneously taste sour, sweet, salty, bitter, and hot. All but 1 of the more than 20 schisandra species are native to eastern Asia; the oddball is a seldom-seen vine that grows in the southeastern United States and is occasionally cultivated as an ornamental. In Asia, the leaves and berries are consumed as food, and herbal preparations are used as all-purpose tonics.

Therapeutic Uses:
🌿🌿 Hepatitis, paralysis, Parkinson's disease, psychosis, stroke.

🌿 Ataxia (a muscular disorder with jerky, irregular movements), cancer, chemotherapy, colds, coughing, depression, fatigue, labor, Ménière's disease, senility, stress, thirst.

▦ Folk uses: Asthma, diarrhea, impotence, insomnia, kidney disease, neurasthenia, urinary excess.

Medicinal Properties:
Traditional Chinese physicians recommend schisandra in much the same way they recommend ginseng—as a general tonic and adaptogen that seems to normalize whatever is out of whack in the body. Research, both clinical and in the lab, backs up some of their claims. Lignans in the plant encourage the revival of liver cells damaged by alcohol, toxic substances, and viral hepatitis. The phytochemicals also improve reflexes, fine coordination, concentration, blood pressure, and physical stamina. Two substances, schisanhenol and schisandrin B, have been shown to protect the brains of lab rats from oxidative stress.

Dosage Options:
Two hundred fifty to 500 milligrams once or twice a day, ½ to 2½ teaspoons of a liquid extract daily, 1 teaspoon of the fresh fruit every day, or ½ to 1 teaspoon of schisandra tincture three times a day.

Safety Rating: 1

Precautions:
A few people might notice some indigestion or itchiness. In a few instances, schisandra might suppress appetite.

SCOTCH BROOM (Cytisus scoparius; Sarothamnus scoparius)

See "Broom" on page 52.

SENNA (Cassia, various species)

What It Is:
In the dry lands of eastern and northern Africa grows a small shrub with flattened pealike pods, delicate yellow flowers, and a powerful purgative punch. Beginning in the ninth century, first the Middle East and then the rest of the world learned of senna's dramatic laxative ability. Several species exist, cultivated commercially in India and various Middle Eastern nations. Many wild senna species contain the same active ingredients.

Therapeutic Uses:
🌿🌿 Constipation.
🌿 Dysentery, ringworm.
▨ Folk uses: Dermatitis, fever, gonorrhea, hemorrhoids, indigestion, wounds.

Medicinal Properties:
Senna is perhaps the brawniest of the herbal bowel boosters. Others include aloes, cascara sagrada, and rhubarb (see "Aloes" on page 29, "Cascara Sagrada" on page 63, and "Rhubarb" on page 185). The strong anthraquinone presence interacts with bacteria in the digestive tract to create a chemical that provokes intestinal contractions.

Prescription Counterparts:
Like cascara sagrada, senna is an active ingredient in many brand-name laxatives (such as Ex-Lax). Why bother with a bunch of fillers, flavorings, and a trademark when you can use a natural substance?

Dosage Options:
When constipated, 50 milligrams of a standardized supplement once or twice a day, ⅛ to ½ teaspoon of a liquid leaf extract daily, or 3 to 6 pods steeped in a cup of warm water every 6 to 12 hours. Senna's seedpods possess more constipation-relieving might than do its leaves, but leaf formulations are deemed safer. To reduce the likelihood of intestinal pain when taking senna, mix it with ginger, cloves, or mint.

Safety Rating: 1

Precautions:
Any laxative, whether from nature or a test tube, is a last-resort, short-term treatment for constipation—a consideration only when a high-fiber diet fails. (For good

sources of natural fiber, see "Oats" on page 159 and "Psyllium" on page 178.) Try senna if the more gentle cascara sagrada doesn't work. Senna seems to be a stronger, more dependable laxative, but it's also more likely to lead to dependency and other problems, such as cramping and loss of potassium.

Don't take senna for more than a week or so. Your body could end up relying on it to contract your bowels, ultimately worsening the original constipation problem. Don't take the herb if you have colitis, Crohn's disease, hemorrhoids, a kidney problem, a bad appendix, or any abdominal pain of unknown origin. Don't take it if you're expecting or nursing a baby. The active compounds could show up in your breast milk. Ingesting senna or any other anthraquinone-containing substance could cause additional problems. Some studies say that extended use is toxic and may promote tumor growth. According to German research, long-term use increases the risk of colon cancer, although this carcinogenic effect has been questioned by other researchers.

SHEPHERD'S PURSE *(Capsella bursa-pastoris)*

What It Is:
The seedpods that emerge from the plant's tiny white flowers look somewhat like the leather satchels in which ancient shepherds carried food, hence the common name of this little mustard-family member. Shepherd's purse—with its ground-hugging, sometimes dandelion-like leaves and central stem or two that might grow up to a foot or so tall—is native to southern Europe and western Asia. But thanks to the thousands of seeds in those pods, it has become established all over the world, including North America.

Therapeutic Uses:
🌿🌿 Burns, cardiac insufficiency, excessive menstruation, heart disease, irregular heartbeat, nosebleeds, premenstrual tension, wounds.
🌿 Inflammation, labor, mucous membrane inflammation, nervousness, tumors, ulcers.
▦ Folk uses: Bloody urine, cystitis, diarrhea, dysentery, fever, headache, hemorrhage, hemorrhoids, menstrual pain, urinary tract infections.

Medicinal Properties:
Shepherd's purse is nature's styptic, used for hundreds of years to halt both internal and external bleeding, whether from a wound, hemorrhoids, or menstruation. Research confirms that an extract of the whole herb does hasten coagulation and constrict blood vessels. At the same time, it also allows coronary arteries to expand and improves blood flow to the heart. It might make your cheeks rosy, too.

Dosage Options:
One-quarter to 1 teaspoon of a liquid extract every day, 20 to 30 drops of a tincture two or three times a day, or 1 teaspoon of the dried herb in a cup of hot water two to four times a day. For cuts and nosebleeds, apply the tea or the liquid extract topically.

Safety Rating: 2

Precautions:
In reasonable amounts, none reported, although given its effect on menstruation, you might want to avoid it if you're pregnant. Because of the herb's oxalate content, you probably shouldn't take it if you have kidney problems or stones. Some observers suggest that shepherd's purse might interact with heart-related medications. Large doses may cause heart palpitations or sedation. Ridiculously huge toxic doses can impair breathing to the point of causing respiratory paralysis and death. Internal bleeding, perhaps manifested as blood in the urine or stool, may occur. If so, consult your doctor immediately.

SIBERIAN GINSENG *(Eleutherococcus senticosus)*

See "Ginseng, Oriental" on page 115.

SKULLCAP *(Scutellaria lateriflora)*

What It Is:
Found in damp woods and swamplands in eastern North America, this plant was used in the late 1700s as a cure for rabies, hence one of its common names, mad dog weed. The claims were later discounted, and herbalists concentrated on the plant's value as a tranquilizer. Skullcap is so named because its two-lobed flowers, which range in color from purple and blue to pink and white, somewhat resemble a military helmet that early American settlers wore. The root of a related species, Baikal skullcap *(S. baicalensis)*, is native to China and is used in traditional Chinese medicine to relieve colds, fever, high blood pressure, and insomnia, among other problems.

Therapeutic Uses:
🐦 Blood clots, stroke, thrombosis.
▦ Folk uses: Addictions, alcoholism, anxiety, childbirth (afterbirth removal), chorea (involuntary spasms of the face and limbs), colds, convulsions, epilepsy, headache, hysteria, insomnia, menstrual pain, nervous tension, rabies, stress.

Medicinal Properties:
Though insufficiently researched, skullcap has shown therapeutic promise against strokes and nervous disorders. In clinical trials involving a total of 634 people with cerebral embolism (blood clot), cerebral thrombosis, or stroke-induced paralysis, an extract of scutellarin, one of the plant's active compounds, improved blood flow for more than 88 percent of the participants, whether the substance was ingested or injected. Other limited research has verified skullcap's ability to quell spasms and to sedate.

Dosage Options:
Eight hundred fifty to 1,290 milligrams two or three times a day, ½ to 1 teaspoon of a liquid extract or tincture, or 1 to 2 teaspoons of the dried herb steeped in a cup of hot water up to three times a day. Select a high-quality, reputable product with an assurance that it contains only *Scutellaria*. In the past, real skullcap was often adulterated with *Teucrium canadense*, or pink skullcap. A related species, *T. chamaedrys*, or germander, has been identified as a cause of liver problems (see "Precautions.")

Safety Rating: 2

Precautions:
In normal amounts, authentic *Scutellaria* is not toxic. Overdoses of skullcap tincture may cause confusion, giddiness, stupor, twitching, and seizures. Because of the plant's traditional use to encourage menstruation and help remove afterbirth, you might want to avoid skullcap if you're pregnant. Perhaps the most important cautionary note is to get authentic *Scutellaria* that has not been cut with herbs in the *Teucrium* genus, one of which is called pink skullcap. Another, germander, reportedly causes hepatitis and liver damage.

SKUNK CABBAGE *(Symplocarpus foetidus)*

What It Is:
This is one of the most appropriately named plants in all of botany. Its leaves really look like cabbage leaves, and all parts of the plant really stink. It is found in damp woods throughout the northern and central United States. You'll know it when you smell it, and just touching it can make some people itchy.

Therapeutic Uses:
▓ Folk uses: Arthritis, asthma, bronchitis, convulsions, coughing, cramps, epilepsy, itching, migraine, toothache, whooping cough, wounds.

Medicinal Properties:
Little research has been conducted on skunk cabbage. Herbalists claim that it quiets muscle spasms, calms you down, breaks up bronchial congestion, and encourages

excretion of excess fluids. Skunk cabbage is, at best, a last resort for relief of migraines.

Dosage Options:
One-eighth to ¼ teaspoon of a liquid root extract, ½ to 1 teaspoon of a root tincture, or ½ to 1 gram of powdered root as a tea or in some honey three times a day. Heat destroys the nasty taste and odor.

Safety Rating:
Don't take it.

Precautions:
Touching the plant can cause skin blisters and nagging itchiness. Don't use skunk cabbage if you have a kidney problem. Taking too much might upset your stomach or make you vomit.

SLIPPERY ELM *(Ulmus rubra)*

What It Is:
On the inside of the rough, reddish brown bark of this native North American tree is a natural medicine with a long, successful history that even the FDA can't deny. Native Americans used slippery elm bark to heal both inside and out, making poultices to treat skin injuries of all sorts and brewing teas to assuage upset stomachs and inflamed tissues. Early settlers followed suit, adding to the list the treatment of gunshot wounds by the time of the American Revolution.

Therapeutic Uses:
🌿🌿 Coughing, gastritis, inflammation, intestinal disease, oral inflammation, sore throat.
🌿 Boils, burns, cold sores, colitis, Crohn's disease, dermatitis, diarrhea, indigestion, sores, stomach problems, ulcers, wounds.
▨ Folk uses: Abscesses, colds, cuts, dysentery, pleurisy.

Medicinal Properties:
The tree's inner bark contains a copious amount of mucilage, a spongy, gummy, even slippery fiber that soothes inflamed, irritated mucous membranes from the inside of your mouth all the way through the rest of your gastrointestinal tract.

Dosage Options:
Six hundred eighty to 1,000 milligrams of a standardized supplement daily, 1 to 3 teaspoons of the powdered herb in a tea up to three times a day, 1 teaspoon of a liquid extract or tincture three times a day, ¼ to ½ cup of fresh bark daily, or 2 to 4 teaspoons of dried bark daily.

Safety Rating: 3

Precautions:

None reported. Slippery elm is safer than coffee. Don't take it with any medications; the mucilage could impede or delay absorption. Some people might be allergic to the tree's pollen.

SOYBEAN *(Glycine max)*

What It Is:

Flour, milk, miso, imitation meat, tempeh, tofu, hydrolyzed vegetable protein, a salty sauce, even printers' inks—some say soy is the world's most versatile food. A member of the bean family—with white pealike flowers that are followed by hairy, bean-containing pods—soy was named one of the five sacred crops in an ancient Chinese medical text more than 2,000 years before the birth of Christ. Its healthful reputation, whether fully deserved or not, has been growing ever since.

Therapeutic Uses:

🌿🌿 High cholesterol.

🌿 Dandruff, endometriosis, hepatitis, lack of appetite, menopause, osteoporosis.

▦ Folk use: Stomach disease.

Medicinal Properties:

Because it contains plant estrogens called isoflavones, soy has been touted far and wide as a natural treatment for and preventive of menopause-related problems and hormone-fueled cancers. In addition, the phospholipids (lecithin and phosphatidylcholine) extracted from soybeans guard the liver and help improve cholesterol levels.

Medicinal Properties for Natural Estrogens

Genistein, daidzein, and the other phytoestrogens in soy are the botanical equivalents of the human female hormones, but much weaker, working in the body much like estrogen and progesterone. When the body's natural concentrations of these hormones decline, phytoestrogens help make up for the deficit, easing menopausal symptoms such as hot flashes, night sweats, and vaginal dryness and perhaps alleviating premenstrual difficulties such as cramping and irritability. The isoflavones also may offer relief for the pain, swelling, nausea, and bleeding of endometriosis.

Phytoestrogens also play a role in inactivating the more harmful forms of human estrogens and estrogen-like pollutants. Certain estrogen metabolites, industrial estrogen chemicals, and synthetic prescription estrogen replacements all have been associated with a higher risk for cancer. But the phytoestrogens prevent the harmful forms from locking onto cellular receptors and doing their damage. Genistein also inhibits the process (called angiogenesis) in which malignant cells trigger blood vessel formation to feed tumor growth.

Although soybeans have monopolized the female phytochemical spotlight, they are by no means the only source or the best source of plant estrogens. Red clover, kudzu, and perhaps flaxseed (see "Red Clover" on page 182, "Kudzu" on page 136, and "Flax" on page 104) all have as good or better concentrations. Many species of clover, in fact, have a better array of phytoestrogens. Foods that have much more genistein (though less daidzein) include yellow split peas, lima beans, red kidney beans, red lentils, black-eyed peas, mung beans, and fava beans. Pinto beans have almost as much genistein and daidzein as soy.

Medicinal Properties for Phospholipids

The liver and cardiovascular system benefit from the oily lecithin and phosphatidylcholine extracted from soybeans and soy seeds. Lecithin is an emulsifier; it breaks down fats, allowing the body to absorb and metabolize cholesterol better. A number of studies have shown that high-soy diets and lecithin supplements lower triglycerides and low-density lipoprotein (LDL) cholesterol, both of which figure into hardening of the arteries, while maintaining a good level of heart-helpful high-density lipoprotein (HDL) cholesterol. Phosphatidylcholine seems to guard the liver from free radical fatty damage and hasten the regeneration of its tissues.

Prescription Counterparts:

The 300 milligrams or so of isoflavone phytoestrogens in 1 cup of soybeans may provide the menopausal relief of one tablet of conjugated estrogens (Premarin).

Dosage Options:

Feel free to eat soy dishes as often as you want. In supplement form, an option is 1 to 3 grams of soy phospholipids containing at least 73 to 79 percent phosphatidylcholine daily.

Safety Rating: 3

Precautions:

None reported. A few people might experience gastric complaints, including loose stools or diarrhea.

SPEARMINT *(Mentha spicata)*

What It Is:

This member of the mint family is full of clonally reproduced hybrids, many difficult to distinguish from one another. And without spearmint, we wouldn't have the stronger-tasting peppermint, which is a hybrid of spearmint and watermint. Peppermint and spearmint both have serrated leaves and lilac or pinkish flowers. Peppermint usually has a longer leaf stalk; botanists call its leaf a petiolate leaf. Spearmint typically has a shorter leaf stalk or no stalk at all, a feature that botanists call a sessile leaf. If you keep in mind that *P* stands for peppermint and petiolate and that *S* stands for spearmint and sessile, it might be easier for you to distinguish between the two.

Therapeutic Uses:

Colds, cramps, gas, gastric disease, headache, indigestion, intestinal disease, stomachache.

Folk uses: Cancer, coughing, depression, diarrhea, fever, nausea.

Medicinal Properties:

Menthol is one of the major medicinal compounds in spearmint, peppermint, and many other members of the mint family. Peppermint usually has a better concentration of this phytochemical than spearmint (see "Peppermint" on page 168).

Dosage Options:

One to 2 tablespoons of the dried herb in a cup of hot water several times a day.

Safety Rating: 3

Precautions:

None reported, but see the precautions under "Peppermint" on page 170.

STEVIA *(Stevia rebaudiana)*

What It Is:

First there were cyclamates. Then there was saccharin. Next came aspartame. And now, in just the past few years, we have acesulfane-K and sucralose. Throughout America's expensive, never-ending quest for a low-calorie artificial substitute for sugar, few have considered the natural alternative: an obscure plant from Paraguay. The active phytochemical in the serrated leaves of stevia, or sweet herb as the locals call it, is at least a hundred times sweeter than sugar. Some 200 or so species of stevia grow throughout Central and South America, but none apparently is as sweet as this one.

Therapeutic Uses:

Diabetes, obesity.

Medicinal Properties:

Stevia isn't just a calorie-free sugar substitute. In one small study, a liquid leaf extract of stevioside, the active component, markedly lowered blood sugar levels for 16 healthy adults, suggesting a possible therapeutic use for people with diabetes.

Dosage Options:

With a beverage, up to 57 milligrams of a standardized extract containing 85 percent steviocides. To sweeten foods and drinks, add just a pinch of stevia powder.

Precautions:

If you have diabetes, keep a closer watch on your blood sugar if you use this herb. Some people don't like the aftertaste; others say that it's not as unpleasant as that of saccharin. Very limited research indicates that stevia might have some contraceptive effects, so you probably shouldn't take it if you're expecting or trying to become pregnant.

STINGING NETTLE *(Urtica dioica)*

See "Nettle" on page 157.

STONEROOT *(Collinsonia canadensis)*

What It Is:

The root looks like a stone, and the plant traditionally has been used to treat stones, whether in the kidneys, bladder, or urinary tract—thus the common name of this toothy-leaved, yellow-flowered perennial that grows wild in eastern and central North America. Although it looks like a nettle, it's a member of the mint family, but not as consistently aromatic. It may smell like lemon.

Therapeutic Uses:

🍂 Bladder disease, intestinal disease, stomach disease.

▦ Folk uses: Bladder stones, bruises, burns, calculus (calcified deposits or formations on the teeth or anywhere in the body), diarrhea, dropsy, hemorrhoids, kidney stones or disease, laryngitis, lithuria (excessive uric acid), sores, sprains, wounds.

Medicinal Properties:

Little research exists to support stoneroot's time-honored use against kidney and bladder stones.

Dosage Options:

One-quarter to 1 teaspoon of a liquid root extract, ½ to 2 teaspoons of stoneroot tincture, or 1 to 4 grams of the dried root in a tea three times a day.

Safety Rating: 2

Precautions:

Don't ingest too much. Overdoses can irritate the lining of your gut, causing nausea, intestinal pain, dizziness, and painful, decreased urination.

SUMA *(Pfaffia paniculata)*

What It Is:
Here's a plant with virtually no folk history, medicinal or otherwise. Nearly 40 years ago, this clambering, nondescript member of the pigweed family (a close kin of amaranth) didn't even have a popular name. Since then, some supplement promoters have created a small body of folklore claiming that the Xingu tribe of Mato Grosso, Brazil, has used suma root as a ginsenglike tonic for at least 300 years. This supposed heritage somehow escaped even one mention in a highly trusted six-volume study of useful Brazilian plants, as well as diligent investigations by other researchers. Believe it if you wish, but chances are you're getting a pigweed in a poke.

Therapeutic Uses:
▨ "Folk" uses: Cancer, diabetes, Epstein-Barr virus, fatigue, menopause, stress.

Medicinal Properties:
Brazilian ginseng? Baloney. Limited Japanese test tube experiments have identified some minor anticancer activity for suma.

Dosage Options:
Five hundred twenty to 1,040 milligrams of the capsulated supplement twice a day or 500 to 1,000 milligrams of the dried herb two or three times a day.

Safety Rating: 2

Precautions:
None reported, other than the fact that suma almost certainly won't do much, good or bad.

SUNDEW *(Drosera, various species)*

What It Is:
A predatory kin of Venus's-flytrap, sundew sits inconspicuously in or along eastern and central North American peat bogs, a ground-hugging whorl of miniature spatula-shaped leaves covered with sticky reddish hairs at the bottom of its long, flower-topped stem. When an unwary insect alights on a gluey leaf, it cannot get off, and then the plant springs into action, secreting a protein-dissolving (proteolytic) juice to digest the bug.

Therapeutic Uses:
✿✿ Asthma, bronchitis, coughing, whooping cough.
✿ Bunions, corns, laryngitis, leishmaniasis, ulcers, warts.
▨ Folk uses: Gastritis, hardening of the arteries.

Medicinal Properties:
The plant's phytochemicals—including plumbagin, carboxy-oxy-napthoquinones, and that insect-eating proteolytic enzyme—aid better breathing by quieting bronchial spasms, helping break up congestion, and soothing irritated mucous membranes. In small amounts, plumbagin revs up the immune system a little, too. It also fights bacterial, viral, and fungal infections, including some of the bacteria involved in laryngitis. Protein-dissolving and germ-killing actions come into play when sundew is applied topically to corns, bunions, and warts.

Prescription Counterparts:
According to German research, sundew compares quite favorably to codeine as a cough suppressant, working for about 90 percent of the people who try it.

Dosage Options:
One-eighth to ½ teaspoon of a liquid leaf extract, ⅛ to ¼ teaspoon of a tincture, or 1 to 2 grams of dried leaves in a cup of hot water three times a day.

Precautions:
None reported, although the plumbagin may be an irritant to some people.

SWEET ANNIE *(Artemisia annua)*

What It Is:
To the eye, sweet Annie's silhouette looks somewhat like asparagus. But its scent is quite distinctive—pleasing to some, irritating to others. In China, it's known as *qing hao;* elsewhere, people know it as annual wormwood or wormweed, which befits a member of the wormwood genus. Sweet Annie's flowers and fruit are multitudinous but so small that they're almost impossible to see. The multitude of flowers produce a multitude of seeds, which has allowed the plant to spread from its native Asia and northern Europe to virtually all parts of the temperate and subtropical world.

Therapeutic Uses:
🌿🌿 Colds, flu, malaria (prevention and treatment), lupus.
🌿 Abscesses, boils, diarrhea, dysentery, fever, gas, infections, leishmaniasis.
▦ Folk uses: Night sweats.

Medicinal Properties:
Sweet Annie boasts at least a half dozen antiviral phytochemicals that fight intestinal parasites. In both laboratory and clinical experiments, its artemisinin has displayed a discriminating, selective, immune-suppressing activity that has some promise against lupus.

Prescription Counterparts:
Extracts of sweet Annie may be better than the prescription drug chloroquine (Aralen) for preventing certain types of malaria and treating fevers and other symptoms of a malarial infection.

Dosage Options:
One and one-half to 2½ tablespoons of a liquid extract daily (more for malaria or lupus) or 50 milligrams of an artemisinin extract for every 2.2 pounds of body weight for 3 days. For lupus, try 300 milligrams of an artemisinin extract or 1 to 1½ ounces of the fresh or dried herb daily for 50 days.

Safety Rating: 2

Precautions:
Sweet Annie may cause a rash, watery eyes, or another allergic reaction.

TEA *(Camellia sinensis)*

What It Is:
Ours is a world divided by color: black versus green. Most of the Western world drinks black tea; much of Asia, the Middle East, and northern Africa drinks green tea. Same shrubby evergreen plant, same hairy ovate leaves, but a different color because of different processing—and, apparently, a different impact on health, again because of the processing. To make green tea, the plant's leaves are steamed and then dried. That's about the extent of it. For black tea, the leaves are dried, rolled, fermented, and roasted. The more extensive handling, heating, and exposure to air changes black tea's chemical composition, reducing some of the medicinal qualities of a main phytochemical group called the polyphenols.

Therapeutic Uses:
🌿🌿 Cavities.
🌿 Alzheimer's disease, arthritis, asthma, cancer (especially colon, liver, lung, pancreas, skin, stomach, and throat), colds, colitis, coughing, diarrhea, dysentery, gum bleeding and disease, headache, heart disease, hemorrhage, high cholesterol, high

triglycerides, infections, inflammation, obesity, polyps, stroke, sunburn, ulcers, wrinkles.

▨ Folk uses: High blood pressure, nausea, stomach disease.

Medicinal Properties:

The better-retained phytochemical complement makes green tea a notable contribution to good health, particularly dental health and prevention of cancer, according to a large, growing body of research. In addition to several antibacterial compounds that fight germs and infections, the polyphenols prevent plaque from building up on your teeth, making green tea excellent protection against cavities and gum disease. (It even contains a bit of fluoride.)

The polyphenols (a large group of phytochemicals that includes epigallocatechin gallate, proanthocyanidins, catechin, and epicatechin, among others) are muscular antioxidants—stronger than vitamins C and E, according to laboratory studies. They also pump up the muscles' own antioxidant enzymes (such as glutathione) and interfere with the creation of cancer-causing nitrosamines that we ingest in such nitrite-laced foods as cured meats. It's no wonder, then, that studies comparing green tea consumption to cancer rates in Japan and China have connected a higher consumption of the minimally processed leaves with a far lower incidence of malignancies.

Tea, whether green or black, contains caffeine. For a review of that phytochemical's therapeutic powers, see "Coffee" on page 78.

Dosage Options:

You already know how to use a tea bag. For loose tea, steep 1 to 2 teaspoons in a cup of hot water and drink up to three times a day. Supplementally, you'll see different polyphenol calculations depending on the brand. Daily options include 100 to 200 milligrams of a green tea supplement standardized for 50 percent polyphenols or 150 to 400 milligrams of polyphenols.

Safety Rating: 2

Precautions:

Green tea and black tea are just as safe as coffee and pose no additional threat. As with coffee, drinking too much tea can cause gastric upset, irritability, jitteriness, and insomnia. Some herbalists claim that green tea, despite its caffeine content, doesn't jangle your nerves as much as black tea, coffee, or cola. (For a discussion of possible problems associated with ingesting too much caffeine, see "Coffee" on page 78.)

TEA TREE *(Melaleuca alternifolia)*

What It Is:

Blame Captain Cook for any confusion between what we know as tea and this diminutive myrtle-family tree whose leaf oil is one of our best natural antiseptics. The aromatic tea tree genus, *Melaleuca,* though not quite as diverse in Australia as the related *Eucalyptus* genus, is another group of species that are difficult to distinguish from one another. In documenting and recounting his exploits in the late 1700s, Cook made reference to the "tea plant," which the ship's crew used to counteract the astringency of a spruce-based beer. Early Aussie settlers also used the tree's grasslike leaves to brew a tea, further entrenching the name. Tea tree, native to the northeastern coast of New South Wales in Australia but also grown elsewhere, is in no way related to what we call tea. It's more akin to the best antiseptics in health care.

Therapeutic Uses:

🍃 Acne, athlete's foot, boils, bunions, calluses, colds, corns, cystitis, dermatitis, fungal infections (including nails), sores, vaginitis, wounds, yeast infections.

▩ Folk uses: Arthritis, bruises, bug bites, burns, dandruff, headache, lice, muscle pain, sunburn, toothache, varicose veins, warts.

Medicinal Properties:

Terpenes and other phytochemicals in tea tree oil are powerful antiseptics and fungus killers that are readily absorbed by the skin. The oil has been successfully put to the test in clinical studies against acne, boils, foot odor, and toenail fungus. It also hastens the healing of corns, calluses, and bunions.

Prescription Counterparts:

For disinfecting a cut or a scrape, tea tree oil is just as good as two old-time standbys—merbromin (Mercurochrome) and iodine. For a vaginal yeast infection, some research shows that tea tree oil is just as good as the prescription drugs nystatin (Mycostatin) and clotrimazole (Lotrimin).

Tea tree oil also works just as well as products that contain benzoyl peroxide (such as Oxy 10) against inflamed acne, but with fewer side effects such as dryness, stinging, and redness. Benzoyl peroxide works better on noninflamed acne, though.

Dosage Options:

Never ingest tea tree oil; it's best reserved for topical treatment. The straight, full-power oil is your best medicinal bet, but start off with a diluted preparation just in case you're sensitive to it (see "Precautions").

Mix some tea tree oil with an equal amount of vegetable oil or water, then apply it to your skin. For dandruff, put a couple of drops in your favorite shampoo.

Safety Rating: 2

Precautions:
For certain people, particularly if they have sensitive skin, tea tree oil could be irritating, especially if applied undiluted. Some cautious commentators say that it will exacerbate eczema, whether diluted or not. Other experts say that despite its effectiveness against candidas, tea tree oil should be used only as a last resort against vaginal infections.

THYME *(Thymus vulgaris)*

What It Is:
Thyme is bravery, valor, and derring-do, at least as far as the ancient Greeks were concerned. The herb's name comes from *thumus,* a Greek word meaning "courage." You don't need to be very courageous, however, to try some thyme in the kitchen. Its aroma and taste are culinary staples of meats, salads, sauces, and soups. The perennial, with its tiny leaves and tiny, whitish pink flowers, grows readily across North America, but the plant originated in the southern Mediterranean.

Therapeutic Uses:
🌿🌿 Bronchitis, coughing, mucous membrane inflammation, respiratory disease, whooping cough.
🌿 Alzheimer's disease, arthritis, athlete's foot, bad breath, bed-wetting, cancer, cavities, colds, colic, colitis, congestion, cramps, dermatitis, fungal infections, gas, gingivitis, hair loss, indigestion, inflammation, intestinal disease, laryngitis, lice, menstrual pain, muscle pain, nail infections, nerve pain, scleroderma, sore throat, stomach disease, tonsillitis, ulcers, vulva disease, worms.
▦ Folk uses: Asthma, bruises, depression, diarrhea, fatigue, fever, gastritis, lack of appetite, premenstrual tension, sprains, stress.

Medicinal Properties:
Thyme has long been dispensed to facilitate breathing, and science has since backed up the traditional use. Thymol, carvacrol, other components of the essential oil, and flavonoids all are good for breaking up congestion, stopping coughing, taming bronchial spasms, and stimulating respiration. The herb's oils also settle the stomach and kill germs and fungi.

Dosage Options:
One teaspoon of thyme syrup several times a day, ½ to 1 teaspoon of a tincture three times a day, ½ to 1 teaspoon of a liquid extract daily, or 1 teaspoon of the dried herb in a cup of hot water up to three times a day.

Safety Rating: 3

Precautions:

None reported. Don't ingest the volatile oil straight. For some sensitive people, toothpastes containing thyme (check the labels) might cause cracking at the corners of the mouth or inflame the tongue.

TOMATO *(Lycopersicon esculentum)*

What It Is:

Soup, juice, sauce—tomato is many things, including a clambering, scented annual whose vine, as anyone who's ever walked through a garden on a summer day knows, often needs to be tied to a stake to keep those juicy orbs off the ground. The one thing a tomato is not, technically speaking, is a vegetable. Whether red, orange, or yellow; plum-shaped, pear-shaped, or globular, the "love apple" is a fruit. Even more technically, it's a berry.

Therapeutic Uses:

☙ Asthma, athlete's foot, cancer, cataracts, diabetes, high blood pressure, high cholesterol, prostate enlargement (benign).

Folk uses: Arthritis, boils, burns, chills, colds, eye inflammation, flu, hangover, heart disease, hemorrhoids, indigestion, inflammation, lack of appetite, palpitations, ringworm, sore throat, urinary pain or problems, worms, yellow fever.

Medicinal Properties:

Tomatoes are juicy globes of antioxidant health, courtesy of their beta-carotene, vitamin C, and lycopene, a relative newcomer to scientific study. Lycopene, perhaps one of the strongest oxidation fighters among the carotenoids, shows much promise against several cancers, including those of the bladder, breast, cervix, and prostate. It also helps check cholesterol accumulation. Seven other phytochemicals in tomatoes, including gamma-aminobutyric acid (GABA), work to control high blood pressure.

Dosage Options:

Let tomatoes be one of the five servings of vegetables or fruits that you should eat every day. You also may find lycopene supplements at the health food store. Check the label for recommended dosages.

Safety Rating: 3

Precautions:

The leaves are poisonous. Some say that green tomatoes aren't all that healthful either, although all the southerners who have eaten fried green tomatoes certainly don't seem to have suffered any ill effects. Green tomatoes do not, however, contain lycopene, which gives tomatoes their red color.

TURMERIC (Curcuma longa)

What It Is:

It's yellow—so yellow that stains from ground turmeric are almost impossible to remove. It's also tasty—so tasty that you're not likely to forget your first turmeric-tinged curry dish. Even that mustard in your refrigerator would be somewhat less golden and tasty without this herb. A kin of cardamom, ginger, and zedoary (see "Cardamom" on page 61, "Ginger" on page 110, and "Zedoary" on page 234), turmeric—its wide, foot-long, lilylike leaves and yellow to yellowish white flowers— is native to India, Bangladesh, China, and Java and has been introduced to Latin America and other tropical lands. But its medicinal and culinary value is in the root—or, to be technically correct, the rhizome (the belowground part of the stem), which is dried and ground into the spice.

Therapeutic Uses:

🌿🌿 Gallbladder problems, hepatitis, indigestion, infections, lack of appetite, scabies.

🌿 Alzheimer's disease, arthritis, asthma, athlete's foot, boils, bunions, bursitis, cancer (especially breast and colon), cataracts, colic, dermatitis, diarrhea, eczema, fibrosis, gallstones, gas, hardening of the arteries, heart disease, high cholesterol, high triglycerides, inflammation, intestinal pain, irritable bowel syndrome, jaundice, lack of menstruation, lymph gland problems, menstrual pain, morning sickness, pain, psoriasis, sprains, ulcers, wounds, yeast infections.

▦ Folk uses: Bruises, childbirth, eye inflammation, epilepsy, fever, hemorrhage, hemorrhoids, itching, ringworm.

Medicinal Properties:

The curcumin and curcuminoids in turmeric are first-rate arthritis-alleviating anti-inflammatories that also help the gallbladder and liver and provide a defense against cancer. These phytochemicals fight inflammation much like a new class of drugs called cyclooxygenase-2 (COX-2) inhibitors (see "Prescription Counterparts"). These drugs inhibit the body's release of COX-2 prostaglandins, which are secreted in response to various sources of inflammation and swelling. Curcumin and the curcuminoids do not interfere with the body's ability to secrete COX-1 prostaglandins, which are needed for proper blood clotting, among other healthy functions. (Aspirin, by contrast, inhibits both COX-1 and COX-2 prostaglandins, which is why it helps with arthritis but also thins the blood and increases the risk for intestinal bleeding and ulcers.)

Against breast cancer, curcumin, along with the genistein in soy (see "Soybean" on page 204), have been shown to inhibit the formation of cancer in breast tissue. The isolated phytochemicals worked better in tandem than they did individually. In research involving 16 chronic smokers, taking 1,500 milligrams of turmeric daily for 30 days reduced mutagens found in the participants' urine. In animal experiments, curcumins slashed the risk of colon cancer by almost 60 percent. This phytochemical seems to neutralize cancer-causing compounds, stop cancerous changes in the cells, and directly fight substances that enable carcinogens to spread and wreak havoc.

The herb also triggers better bile flow, which helps digest fats and reduces the risk of gallstones. In addition, turmeric generates the secretion of several enzymes that assist the liver in breaking down and metabolizing certain toxic substances. Some of these same phytochemicals inhibit the oxidative damage that allows cholesterol to coagulate and cling to the inside of arteries.

Prescription Counterparts:

Prescription corticosteroids are the "gold standard" for treatment of arthritis, but they bloat the face, cause fluid retention, elevate blood pressure, encourage intestinal bleeding and ulcer formation, and increase the risk of osteoporosis, among other problems.

Vigorously promoted COX-2 drugs such as celecoxib (Celebrex), the top-selling new pharmaceutical of 1999, have been advertised as bringing nonsteroidal anti-inflammatory relief without risk to the stomach and the rest of the gastrointestinal system, but later research indicates that Celebrex does pose problems for people with gastric conditions, particularly by impairing the healing of damaged intestinal linings.

Turmeric/curcumin is about half as effective as corticosteroids, but it doesn't impose any of the side effects noted above. Experiments show that 1,200 milligrams of curcumin a day works as effectively as hydrocortisone acetate (Anusol), indomethacin, and phenylbutazone (Butazone).

Dosage Options:

Four hundred milligrams of a curcumin extract three times a day, 445 milligrams of a standardized supplement two or three times a day, 1 teaspoon of the dried herb in a cup of warm milk daily, 1 teaspoon to 1 tablespoon of a liquid extract divided into several dosages over the course of a day, or ⅛ to ¼ teaspoon of turmeric tincture three times a day. Your body will take up more curcumin if you ingest it with a lot of black pepper. The piperine in pepper improves the body's ability to use turmeric perhaps as much as twentyfold, according to research. Ginger (see "Ginger" on page 110) is a good phytochemical companion, too.

Safety Rating: 3

Precautions:

Few reported with reasonable use. People with a bile duct obstruction probably shouldn't take the herb, and people with gallstones should talk to an herb-savvy physician first. Extremely large doses of curcuminoids could cause ulcers or cancer and reduce the number of red and white corpuscles in the body. If turmeric accounts for 10 percent of your total diet, as it did for some lab rats in one experiment, some of your hair might fall out.

U

UVA URSI *(Arctostaphylos uva-ursi)*

See "Bearberry" on page 35.

V

VALERIAN *(Valeriana officinalis)*

What It Is:
Phu! That's the name the ancient Greeks gave to this long-stemmed perennial. (Nowadays, we'd probably translate the original Greek onomatopoeia as "P-U!") Above ground, the plant is attractive physically and aromatically, with fernlike leaves and fragrant pinkish or white flowers. But below the surface, where the medicine lies, are roots with an earthy, disagreeable smell and taste. The Greeks, beginning with Hippocrates, used valerian roots to help them fall asleep, an application that still holds up under scientific scrutiny. Ironically, what sedates humans supposedly excites cats and mice. Legend has it that the Pied Piper of Hameln did not just toot his flute to drive out the rodents; he baited them with valerian.

Therapeutic Uses:
〜〜〜 Insomnia.
〜〜 Anxiety, nervousness, nervous tension, restlessness, stress.
〜 Acne, depression, epilepsy, exhaustion, fatigue.
▦ Folk uses: Arthritis, cholera, chorea (involuntary spasms of the face and limbs), colic, colitis, cramps, eczema, fever, gum disease, headache, hypochondria, hysteria, indigestion, inflammation, intestinal disease, menstrual pain, migraine, nau-

sea, nerve pain, neuroses, panic, plague, shell shock, skin problems, sores, sore throat, vaginitis, yeast infections.

Medicinal Properties:
We know conclusively that valerian sedates, quiets the central nervous system, and minimizes muscle spasms—just like pharmaceutical tranquilizers. After a few thousand years of use and study, though, we still don't know exactly why. At first, researchers attributed the medicinal effects to just two phytochemical classes, called the valepotriates and the bornyl esters. Now we know that there are several more, including valeranone and the kessyl esters. This is another example of the whole herb being better than the sum of its parts.

Prescription Counterparts:
Combined with St. John's wort, valerian bested diazepam (Valium) in a 2-week trial involving 100 people being treated for anxiety. (Despite the name similarity, Valium is not derived from valerian, nor is there any other relationship between the drug and the herb.) A different double-blind study proved that the herb, this time coupled with hops, was superior to triazolam (Halcion), another benzodiazepine, for relieving sleep disorders. In both studies, the natural remedy worked just as well as the pharmaceutical, but with none of the common side effects—including impairment of mental reactions, upset stomach, dream disturbance or recall, and day-after "hangover"—associated with the habit-forming medications. The demonstrated efficacy and safety have made valerian the active ingredient in dozens of over-the-counter European sleep aids.

Dosage Options:
Three hundred to 500 milligrams of a standardized supplement once a day (or, for insomnia, at bedtime), 1,425 milligrams of an unstandardized supplement three times a day (or, for insomnia, 1,425 to 2,780 milligrams just before turning in), ½ to 1 teaspoon of a root extract or tincture once or more a day, or 1 teaspoon of dried valerian root in a cup of hot water once a day or before bedtime.

Safety Rating: 3

Precautions:
None reported or verified with reasonable use. Very rarely, someone might get an upset stomach or experience a skin reaction. Some observers warn that long-term use might cause headaches, restlessness, insomnia, or heart irregularities.

VERVAIN *(Verbena officinalis)*

What It Is:
It's not mentioned in the Bible, and biblical scholars would dispute the claim, but legend has it that those who retrieved Christ's body from the cross on Calvary used this inconspicuous plant to stop his wounds from bleeding, giving rise to vervain's general reputation as a sacred good luck charm. Witches and warlocks liked to use it, especially in supposed aphrodisiacs, as did herbal physicians, who prescribed it for a whole range of illnesses, particularly colds, gout, and liver problems. An annual with light blue or lilac flowers that grows 1 to 3 feet tall, vervain is indigenous to the Mediterranean but is now a somewhat common weed in temperate areas of North America. It's also cultivated elsewhere in the world, primarily eastern Europe.

Therapeutic Uses:
Breast milk deficiency, coughing, dry mouth, inflammation, pain, sores.

Folk uses: Acne, anemia, arthritis, asthma, bleeding, bruises, colds, cramps, debility, depression, dropsy, erectile dysfunction, fatigue, fever, gout, headache, hepatitis, indigestion, influenza, itchiness, jaundice, kidney disease, liver disease, malaria, melancholy, menopause, menstrual pain, migraine, neurasthenia, neuroses, spleen disease, urinary tract infections, whooping cough, wounds.

Medicinal Properties:
Vervain has helped tamp down inflammation, quiet coughs, and encourage the mouth to water in animal and test tube experiments. It also has increased the secretion of breast milk and stimulated uterine contractions, which may help explain the plant's reputation as an aphrodisiac and its folk uses for menstrual pain and menopause. Either or both of two phytochemicals, aucubin and rosmarinic acid, could be responsible; the research is inconclusive.

Dosage Options:
One-half to 1 teaspoon of a liquid extract three times a day, 1 to 2 teaspoons of a tincture three times a day, or 1 teaspoon of the dried herb steeped in a cup of hot water up to four times a day.

Safety Rating: 2

Precautions:
None reported with reasonable use, although some observers warn that pregnant women should avoid it because of research demonstrating that it can trigger uterine contractions. Large doses might interfere with hormone therapy or blood pressure medications.

W

WHITE HOREHOUND *(Marrubium vulgare)*

What It Is:

Until 1900, horehound, a relatively nonaromatic member of the mint family, was an accepted medicinal in the U.S. Pharmacopeia. The plant, with its furry leaves and tiny whitish flowers, has almost no aroma and tastes rather bitter. It was found in various over-the-counter nostrums, including cough drops, until 1989, when the FDA challenged its use for a supposed lack of efficacy. A year later and a continent away, Germany's Commission E endorsed horehound's folk reputation as an effective treatment for coughing, colds, and indigestion. Decide for yourself.

Therapeutic Uses:

❧❧ Bloating, bronchitis, coughing, gallbladder disease, gas, indigestion, lack of appetite, liver disease.

❧ Colds, diabetes, heart disease, high blood pressure, irregular heart rhythm, laryngitis, respiratory disease, sore throat.

▣ Folk uses: Asthma, diarrhea, intestinal disease, jaundice, menstrual pain, mucous membrane inflammation, skin problems, sores, stomach disease, whooping cough, wounds.

Medicinal Properties:

Studies have demonstrated that horehound breaks up phlegm, relieves bronchial congestion, and triggers bile production. The medicinal chemicals responsible for horehound's expectorant action, marrubiin and marrubinic acid, also help stabilize heart rhythm.

Dosage Options:

One-half to 1 teaspoon of horehound syrup or a liquid extract, 2 to 6 tablespoons of fresh horehound juice, or 1 to 2 grams of the dried herb steeped in a cup of hot water daily.

Safety Rating: 2

Precautions:

Large amounts can act as a laxative. Ingesting as much as five cups of tea, each containing 1 to 2 grams of the herb, might disturb heart rhythm. The plant's juice also might irritate the skin of certain sensitive people.

WHITE WILLOW *(Salix alba)*

What It Is:
Every time you open up the medicine cabinet and reach for an aspirin to relieve a headache, a hangover, or the pain of an arthritic elbow, you owe a big debt to this tree. It's been used to combat pain and treat fevers for some 2,500 years. Some say that meadowsweet (see "Meadowsweet" on page 148) was the first herb from which Bayer, back in the late 1800s, derived its synthetic acetylsalicylic acid—aspirin to us. That may or may not be true, but other members of the 300-strong *Salix* clan—including crack willow *(S. fragilis)*, purple osier *(S. purpurea)*, and violet willow *(S. daphnoides)*—have higher concentrations of this natural pain reliever. The inner bark of the white willow tree, however, is often credited as the original and most frequently used source of it. White willow, with its long, thin, finely serrated leaves, originated in central Asia and Europe but is now naturalized over a good portion of eastern North America, as far north as Nova Scotia and as far south as Georgia.

Therapeutic Uses:
🖝🖝 Pain, rheumatoid arthritis.

🖝 Ankylosing spondylitis (a rheumatoid inflammation of the vertebrae), cataracts, chest pain, colds, corns, diarrhea, fever, gout, headache, heart disease, infections, inflammation, influenza, mucous membrane inflammation, muscle pain, osteoarthritis, poison ivy, skin problems, sprains, toothache, warts.

▦ Folk uses: Bursitis, cancer, earache, obesity, sores.

Medicinal Properties:
The body converts the salicin in white willow (and other species in the willow family) into salicylic acid, the chemical form required to counteract pain, cool inflammation, and deter heart-threatening blood clots. The body also transforms the entirely artificial acetylsalicylic acid in aspirin into salicylic acid. For all practical purposes, then, willow and aspirin are the same.

Prescription Counterparts:
The advent of acetylsalicylic acid sounded the death knell for the use of natural salicin. This is one of the few instances in which a natural medicine is cheaper when synthesized than when extracted from the plant. When Bayer unveiled this product, the company claimed that its invention was easier on the stomach than the "unacetylated" salicin in willow bark. We now know that aspirin also irritates the stomach and encourages ulcers. Indeed, aspirin and other nonsteroidal anti-inflammatory drugs (NSAIDs) kill between 10,000 and 20,000 people annually. Natural salicin may take a little longer to work, herbal authorities concede, but it lasts longer and does not pose as great a risk for gastrointestinal harm.

Don't forget that salicylic acid is also the main ingredient in over-the-counter wart dissolvers and corn removers. You may want to try dissolving an aspirin tablet on that bump or applying a bit of white willow bark instead.

Dosage Options:

One to 2 teaspoons of powdered willow bark steeped in a cup of hot water up to three times a day; 760 to 1,140 milligrams of a willow bark supplement every three hours as needed, up to a daily total of no more than 9,800 milligrams; ¼ to ½ teaspoon of willow bark tincture three times a day; 20 to 40 milligrams of extracted salicin three times a day; ¼ to ¾ teaspoon of a liquid bark extract three times a day; or 1 to 4 teaspoons of fresh willow bark every day.

According to herbal experts, willow tea dilutes salicin's gut-aggravating potential. To further counter possible gastrointestinal problems, you might want to take a licorice extract (see "Licorice" on page 140). Licorice extracts can elevate blood pressure in some people, so you might be better off using a bit of garlic (see "Garlic" on page 106). The beauty of phytochemical combinations (from edible plants that your genes already know) is that they rarely present a peril similar to that of mixing medications.

Safety Rating: 2

Precautions:

If you've been told not to take aspirin, you probably shouldn't take white willow either. Any type of salicylate can interact with alcohol and drugs such as sedatives, barbiturates, and anticoagulants. Huge doses of salicylates can cause nausea, a skin reaction, kidney inflammation, or ringing in the ears. Children who take aspirin-like drugs for colds, chickenpox, and other viral infections run the risk of contracting a liver-damaging, brain-damaging, potentially fatal condition called Reye's syndrome. Salicylates can leach into breast milk, so think twice about using it if you're pregnant or nursing.

WILD CHERRY *(Prunus serotina)*

What It Is:

The white blossoms are gorgeous, the fruit is delicious, and the red-tinged wood makes beautiful furniture. But let's not neglect the utility of the smooth bark of this indigenous North American tree, also called black cherry or, because the fruit can taste a little on the sour side, chokecherry (although those in the know use that name for an even sourer species, *P. virginiana*). Native Americans made a tea from the bark to curtail diarrhea and soothe lung afflictions. The remedy was good enough for early Americans to include wild cherry in many cough elixirs.

Therapeutic Uses:

❧ Bronchitis, cancer, cough, diarrhea, insomnia, intestinal inflammation, pain.

▦ Folk uses: Anxiety, colds, debility, fever, indigestion, labor, lack of appetite, pneumonia, respiratory disease, stress, whooping cough.

Medicinal Properties:
Smith Brothers, Luden's, Vicks, and various other companies had more on their minds than flavor when making wild cherry cough drops. The herb is a decent decongestant that helps curb coughing, settle spasms, break up phlegm, and cool inflammation. It's also slightly sedating—all in all, a nice combination when you're feeling under the weather.

Dosage Options:
One teaspoon of powdered bark steeped in a cup of hot water up to three times a day, ½ to 1 teaspoon of a bark tincture daily, or ½ to 2 teaspoons of a bark syrup every day.

Safety Rating: 2

Precautions:
Though safe in commonly recommended amounts, wild cherry bark is not for long-term use. Unreasonably large doses might include toxic levels of cyanide.

WILD YAM *(Dioscorea villosa)*

What It Is:
This perennial vine is not your Thanksgiving Day sweet potato. It has heart-shaped leaves and a long, knotted, woody rhizome and root with an awful taste that no amount of candying will help. Native Americans used the boiled root to treat morning sickness and facilitate childbirth. Others considered it of some help against arthritis and gastrointestinal woes. Much later, chemists discovered in the root a substance called diosgenin, which can be transformed in the laboratory into sex steroids and corticosteroids. Wild yam grows from New England west to Minnesota and south to Texas. Another species found south of the border and commonly called Mexican yam may yield even more diosgenin than the temperate American vine.

Therapeutic Uses:
🍠 High cholesterol, high triglycerides, intestinal disease, rheumatoid arthritis.
▦ Folk uses: Colic, gallstones, gastritis, hiccups, irritable bowel syndrome, labor, menopause, menstrual pain, morning sickness, muscle pain.

Medicinal Properties:
Much ado has been made about wild yam's early use by pharmaceutical companies to synthesize birth control pills and other steroidal drugs. Marketers claim that the diosgenin in root supplements can elevate levels of testosterone, progesterone, and other hormonal compounds. Scientists can perform the transformation in the laboratory, but the body cannot do it by itself. No studies have proved the supplement suppliers' claims. Not that researchers haven't tried. In one tiny experiment, seven

people took the root for 3 weeks to see if it elevated dehydroepiandrosterone (DHEA), one of the precursor substances that the body uses to make its own hormones. At the end of the experiment, blood readings of DHEA had not changed at all. Researchers did, however, notice a decline in participants' cholesterol levels.

Dosage Options:
Five hundred milligrams of a standardized supplement or 1,000 milligrams of an unstandardized supplement daily, ½ to 1 teaspoon of a liquid root extract daily, ½ teaspoon of a root tincture twice a day, or 1 to 2 teaspoons of fresh root every day. Incidentally, if you want a better source of diosgenin, look to fenugreek (see "Fenugreek" on page 101).

Safety Rating: 3

Precautions:
Large doses could make you vomit or otherwise cause gastric upset. Some preparations of Mexican yam contain additional progesterone to ensure a therapeutic response. New research questions the safety of using extra progesterone to balance estrogen levels.

WITCH HAZEL *(Hamamelis virginiana)*

What It Is:
Widely used by Native Americans for all sorts of skin afflictions, witch hazel remains today almost as common as aspirin in medicine cabinets. There's nothing supernatural about this shrub, except, perhaps, for how its seed capsules eject their contents with a sudden, startling, cracking sound. The *witch,* once spelled "wyche," comes from an old Anglo-Saxon word meaning "bend," a reference to the pliancy of the shrub's branches, which were favorites among dowsers. Witch hazel is a native of eastern and central North America. It doesn't produce its petals, which look somewhat like used yellow twist ties, until after its leaves fall in the autumn. On the East Coast, the flowers sometimes emerge on Halloween, perhaps reinforcing the "witch" connection.

Therapeutic Uses:
🌿🌿 Burns, dermatitis, hemorrhoids, oral inflammation, sore throat, varicose veins, wounds.

🌿 Abrasions, arthritis, asthma, bloody sputum, bruises, bug bites, cholera, colds, Crohn's disease, diarrhea, eczema, gingivitis, herpes, inflammation, intestinal bleeding and inflammation, itchiness, menstrual pain, sores, sunburn, tissue swelling, uterine hemorrhage, vomiting of blood, water retention.

▦ Folk uses: Colitis, coughing, eye inflammation, lung disease, muscle pain.

Medicinal Properties:
The astringent tannins and other phytochemicals in witch hazel counteract pain, soothe, cool, tone blood vessels, and improve circulation—making the herb an all-purpose palliative for everything from abrasions and minor bleeding to varicose veins and most other skin problems. It's notably effective in alleviating hemorrhoid discomfort.

Prescription Counterparts:
Some smart herbal marketer should come up with a product called "Preparation Hamamelis," because witch hazel is a worthy natural alternative to the well-known commercial ointment Preparation H. It once was the active ingredient in another hemorrhoid medication, Tucks. In both cases, it's far less expensive to use a cotton ball dampened with witch hazel.

Dosage Options:
The alcohol distillate available at any supermarket or pharmacy is best reserved for topical use only. Dampen a soft cloth or some cotton with it and put the compress in place. Internal consumption of witch hazel extracts, tinctures, and teas is not recommended (see "Precautions"), although you will find them at health food stores. On the skin, witch hazel tea might not be as dehydrating as the alcohol distillate.

Safety Rating: 2

Precautions:
For external use, none reported, not even during pregnancy, although a few very sensitive people might experience minor skin irritation. Witch hazel extracts and teas shouldn't be ingested because of the herb's high tannin content and the presence, albeit minimal, of safrole, a carcinogen that might contribute to liver damage. Consumption also could cause stomach irritation, nausea, vomiting, diarrhea, or constipation. You should never treat yourself for signs of internal bleeding, such as coughing up blood or blood in the stool. Such symptoms could indicate a serious problem. Consult your doctor.

WOOD BETONY *(Stachys officinalis)*

What It Is:
This mint-family member was revered as a panacea from the days of ancient Greece through the Middle Ages. The Spanish used to say, "He has as many virtues as betony," a great compliment. Native to Europe and Russia, this low-growing perennial sprouts most of its larger leaves near the ground, with much smaller leaves growing along its stalks. These stalks may grow up to 2 feet tall and are topped with whitish, pinkish, or purplish bicolored flowers.

Therapeutic Uses:

🪶 Anxiety, dermatitis, diarrhea, gallbladder problems, gingivitis, headache, indigestion, intestinal inflammation, nerve pain, neuroses, oral inflammation, premenstrual tension, sore throat.

▦ Folk uses: Asthma, bladder stones, bronchitis, coughing, gout, heartburn, kidney stones, lung disease, mucous membrane inflammation, nervousness, stress, wounds.

Medicinal Properties:

Most of wood betony's therapeutic value comes courtesy of its astringent tannins, although Russian researchers have reported finding phytochemicals that reduce inflammation, stimulate the flow of digestion-helping bile, and lower blood pressure.

Dosage Options:

One-half to 1 teaspoon of a liquid extract or 1 to 2 teaspoons of the fresh herb daily.

Safety Rating: 2

Precautions:

None reported.

WORMWOOD *(Artemisia absinthium)*

What It Is:

This herb, which is somewhat woody at the base and has grayish green leaves and clusters of miniature yellow flowers, once had an almost hallowed health-restoring reputation. Native to Europe but now found growing wild from Newfoundland south to Pennsylvania, wormwood was said to counteract poisoning from toadstools and hemlock (as well as the bites of sea dragons); treat liver disease, gout, and kidney stones; dispel intestinal worms; repel fleas, weevils, and other vermin; encourage menstruation; calm the mind and the nerves; and "cure" drunkenness. The latter is a most curious application, given wormwood's ties to the booze business. Brewers used to use it to increase the headiness of beer. Distillers made it the primary constituent of absinthe, an addictive, narcotic nineteenth-century liqueur so notorious for damaging both the brain and the nerves that it was eventually banned (well, almost). The herb also was once known as *wermuth* (preserver of the mind). Change the *w* to a *v*, and you have a liquor that still contains a touch of wormwood.

Therapeutic Uses:

🪶🪶 Gallbladder problems, indigestion, lack of appetite, liver disease.

🪶 Colic, fever, gas, malaria, parasitic infections, roundworm, threadworm, worms.

▦ Folk uses: Anemia, arthritis, bug bites, colds, drunkenness, gastritis, gout, intestinal inflammation, irritable bowel syndrome, kidney stones, lack of menstruation, menstrual pain, poisoning, skin problems, stomachache, stress, wounds.

Medicinal Properties:
The addictive, degenerative influence of absinthe killed wormwood's use as an herbal medicine. In a way, that's too bad, because two of its phytochemicals, absinthin and anabsinthin, do stimulate digestion, and the extract does improve liver and gallbladder function in people with liver disease. It also makes the mouth water and stomach juices flow. Straight thujone, another of the phytochemicals, supposedly is a hallucinogenic brain depressant that inhibits the ability to breathe.

Dosage Options:
One-quarter to ½ teaspoon of a liquid extract daily, 1 teaspoon of the dried herb in a cup of hot water up to three times a day before or after meals, or 10 to 20 drops of wormwood tincture stirred into a glass of water three times a day before meals.

Safety Rating: 1

Precautions:
Not for long-term use, possibly no more than 4 consecutive weeks, if that long. Pregnant women and nursing mothers shouldn't take it at all because of thujone's tendency to provoke uterine contractions. People with ulcers also probably shouldn't use it. Don't exceed dosage recommendations. Excessive consumption could be toxic. Overdoses of thujone can cause insomnia, intestinal cramps, nausea, dizziness, seizures, tremors, brain damage, and ultimately death.

YARROW *(Achillea millefolium)*

What It Is:
This herb was named after the Greek warrior Achilles, who supposedly used yarrow's fernlike leaves to stanch the bleeding of his fellow warriors, hence one of its colorful common names, stanchwort. Long ago, Europeans also called it *Herba militaris,* because they continued to use its broccoli-like clusters of creamy flowers to stop the bleeding of combat injuries. Though native to Europe, you'll find yarrow growing naturally everywhere in North America except the Southwest.

Therapeutic Uses:

☙☙ Gallbladder problems, gastritis, hemorrhage, intestinal bleeding, lack of appetite, liver disease, menstrual pain.

☙ Arthritis, backache, burns, congestion, coughing, diarrhea, fever, infections, inflammation, intestinal disease, nosebleeds, pain, stomach disease, thrombosis, urinary tract infections, wounds.

▦ Folk uses: Colds, colic, high blood pressure, mucous membrane inflammation, rashes, stroke.

Medicinal Properties:

Yarrow helps stop bleeding and counters inflammation and tissue swelling, so it is of some benefit for wounds, especially those that heal slowly. But researchers have focused on other therapeutic qualities of the herb. Some of its phytochemicals ease muscle spasms, making it helpful against menstrual cramps. It also stimulates the gallbladder's release of bile, which improves digestion and eases gastric complaints. Some consider it the poor person's chamomile.

Dosage Options:

One-half to 1 teaspoon of a liquid extract or tincture three times a day, 3 teaspoons of yarrow juice daily, or 1 to 2 teaspoons of the dried herb in a cup of water three or four times a day.

Safety Rating: 2

Precautions:

Certain people may be allergic to yarrow; a few others might get a case of contact dermatitis from it. The herb contains trace amounts of thujone, a phytochemical that, in sufficient amounts, can trigger uterine contractions. For this reason, pregnant women might wish to avoid the herb. Excessive dosages could interfere with or enhance the actions of sedatives, diuretics, blood pressure drugs, and blood thinners.

YELLOW DOCK (Rumex crispus)

What It Is:

Dock is one of our more common weeds, a perennial herb with most of its strap-shaped leaves concentrated at the plant's base over a stout yellowish root. Come summer, yellow dock flowers as it reaches for the sky, growing (in fertile soil) more than 3 feet tall and featuring light brown, buckwheatlike, angular seeds in darker brown envelopes.

Therapeutic Uses:

☙ Constipation, dermatitis, diarrhea, gingivitis, hives and other skin eruptions, infections, intestinal inflammation, psoriasis, ringworm.

Folk uses: Acne, anemia, arthritis, bronchial disease, bruises, burns, eczema, enlarged lymph glands, jaundice, liver inflammation, rhinitis, sores, sore throat, syphilis, tuberculosis, venereal disease.

Medicinal Properties:
Though slightly antibacterial against a few microbes, yellow dock is perhaps most frequently considered a bowel aid that works whichever way you need it. The astringent tannins are of some mild help against diarrhea, while the anthraquinones are gentle laxatives.

Dosage Options:
One-half to 1 teaspoon of a liquid extract three times a day, 1,010 to 1,515 milligrams of a root powder supplement daily, ¼ to ½ teaspoon of dock tincture three times a day, 2 to 4 teaspoons of fresh dock root daily, or 1 to 2 teaspoons of the dried herb steeped in a cup of hot water three or four times a day.

Safety Rating: 2

Precautions:
As with any laxative, yellow dock is not for prolonged use—8 to 10 days at the most. Because of its oxalate content, people with kidney stones should avoid it. Because of the anthraquinones, pregnant women and nursing mothers shouldn't take it either. Anyone with an intestinal illness should think twice, too.

YERBA MANSA *(Anemopsis californica)*

What It Is:
West of the Mississippi and into Mexico, this white-flowered perennial has been used for a broad range of ailments. The "tame herb," as its name translates, grows semiaquatically in salty waters and even warm springs.

Therapeutic Uses:
Fever, insomnia, muscle aches.

Folk uses: Abscesses, arthritis, bronchitis, colds, colic, congestion, consumption, coughing, cystitis, diabetes, fits, flu, gingivitis, gonorrhea, herpes, indigestion, infections, lack of appetite, laryngitis, menstrual pain, mucous membrane inflammation, muscle pain, rectal inflammation, rhinitis, sinus problems, sores, sore throat, stomachache, syphilis, tissue swelling, ulcers, urethritis, vaginal inflammation, water retention.

Medicinal Properties:
Yerba mansa is one of those plants for which there is little scientific evidence to back up its popular use. That doesn't mean it's not beneficial, just that researchers haven't bothered to investigate it. It does appear to relax muscles, calm the central

nervous system, and reduce fevers, at least in part explaining its common use for all the symptoms that accompany colds, flu, and intestinal woes. It also tastes good—a little like cinnamon.

Dosage Options:
One to 2 droppers of a tincture two or three times a day or 4 to 8 grams of dried root daily.

Safety Rating: 1

Precautions:
Because of the lack of scientific information, there's no way to say for sure how safe the herb might be for pregnant women or nursing mothers. The little animal experimentation that has been done suggests that yerba mansa could compound the effects of barbiturates and sedatives.

YERBA SANTA *(Eriodictyon californicum)*

What It Is:
A varnishlike brown resin covers the stem and thick yellowish leaves (which grow up to 6 inches long) of this short evergreen shrub, which sometimes reaches a height of 6 to 8 feet. It grows in clumps, usually on hillsides in California and northern Mexico. Yerba santa once was a popular, bitter-tasting tonic on the West Coast, and people used to smoke its leaves to alleviate asthma.

Therapeutic Uses:
🌢 Allergies, asthma, bronchitis, cancer, colds, cramps, dermatitis, fever, inflammation, poison ivy, respiratory disease, rheumatism, thrush, urinary tract infections, yeast infections.
▦ Folk uses: Arthritis, bruises, colds, coughing, hay fever, pain, tuberculosis, wounds.

Medicinal Properties:
The limited experimentation done on yerba santa indicates that its essential oil can help break up congestion. It also eases inflammation and aids in eliminating excess fluid, both of which help relieve arthritis pain. It displays a little anticancer action, too. Most of its benefits, like those of many others in the citrus family, lie in its aromatic oil.

Dosage Options:
One-half to 1 teaspoon of a liquid herb extract, 10 to 20 drops of a liquid leaf extract, 1 tablespoon of the dried herb in a glass of warm water, or 1 to 2 teaspoons of fresh leaves daily.

Safety Rating: 2

Precautions:
None reported.

YOHIMBE *(Pausinystalia johimbe)*

What It Is:
Inside the bark of this West African tree may be your best natural bet for reversing sexual dysfunction, though at the cost of several side effects. Until the advent of sildenafil citrate (Viagra), the most commonly prescribed drug for erection problems was a pharmaceutical isolation of yohimbe's active phytochemical, yohimbine. Africans have turned to this towering evergreen aphrodisiac for centuries, and Europeans finally took notice in the late 1800s. The whole herb is billed in health food stores not only as a sexual stimulant and erectile aid but also as a muscle-building natural version of the anabolic steroids.

Therapeutic Uses:
〰〰 Erectile dysfunction.
〰 Depression.
▦ Folk uses: Chest pain, exhaustion, feebleness, high blood pressure, low libido (in women).

Medicinal Properties:
For a significant number of the men who try it, yohimbe lives up to its reputation. However, because of its potential side effects, it is one of the rare herbs that's probably safer to use as a prescription drug (see "Prescription Counterparts" and "Precautions"). Early on, a couple of small clinical studies established that yohimbe (the herb, as opposed to yohimbine, the drug alkaloid) enabled about half the participants with psychologically based sexual dysfunction to have an erection. Similarly, it benefited about 40 percent of the men who were unable to achieve erections for physical reasons, such as vascular problems or diabetes. Once the active ingredient was isolated and extracted, almost all the subsequent research concentrated on the pharmaceutical.

Studies have found that yohimbine (the drug) is definitely better than a placebo. In one 10-week effort, almost half of 48 men with psychological-based erectile disorders enjoyed at least some restoration of sexual function. In another trial, lasting a month, 28 of 82 men with erectile disorders reported being able to achieve either full or partial erections. Only a few minor side effects occurred.

Yohimbine is an alpha-adrenergic blocker that allows better blood flow to the genitals, among other physiologic actions. Theoretically, it should work for women as well as for men, because the mechanism of sexual arousal and release is essentially the same in both genders. Anecdotal evidence supports the theory. Its action is apparently unrelated to bolstering the body's production of testosterone, which means it probably is of little value in building bigger muscles.

Prescription Counterparts:
Prescription yohimbine hydrochloride (Yocon, Yohimex, Erex, Aphrodyne) is safer to ingest than supplemental extracts of yohimbe bark. Both can have the same side effects (see "Precautions").

Dosage Options:
The safest dosage is that for yohimbine hydrochloride as prescribed by a doctor. For the over-the-counter herb, you'll find several suggestions on product labels, including 400 to 800 milligrams daily of a standardized supplement containing 8 to 16 milligrams of yohimbine, ½ to 1 teaspoon of a liquid bark extract daily, 5 to 10 drops of yohimbe tincture three times a day, or 1 ounce of dried bark steeped in 2 cups of hot water every day. If you choose the over-the-counter route, you can take yohimbe at any time of day, but the best results might be achieved by taking it an hour or more before engaging in sexual intercourse.

Safety Rating: 1

Precautions:
Both the herbal supplement and the prescription isolate can cause side effects, but the risk is reportedly lower with the drug. In standard dosages (typically 15 to 30 milligrams of pharmaceutical-grade yohimbine daily), those side effects may include anxiety, dizziness, rapid heart rate, blood pressure elevation, blood pressure reduction, insomnia, and nausea. Higher amounts could provoke hallucinations and cause muscular dysfunction. People with liver disease, kidney disease, or a genital infection or inflammation should not use either the herb or the drug. Be particularly wary if you're taking monoamine oxidase inhibitors (MAOIs) or tricyclic antidepressants for depression; the herb can augment the effects of MAOIs, and the medication can send your blood pressure into the stratosphere. As little as 10 milligrams of prescription yohimbine can cause a manic episode in people with the mood swings of bipolar depression.

The connection with blood pressure is contradictory. Some research says that yohimbe will elevate blood pressure; other research suggests that it will depress blood pressure to a possibly dangerous level. No authoritative study has resolved this discrepancy. The herb contains compounds capable of pulling your blood pressure either way. By stimulating blood flow to the genitals, perhaps it draws blood from elsewhere in the body, which might give rise to a low blood pressure reading. But it also is excitatory, which could increase blood pressure.

YUCCA (*Yucca,* various species)

What It Is:
When added to cat food and dog food, extracts of certain yucca species considerably lowered the smell of animal excrement. That's just one of the versatile uses for the several species in this genus of plants that grow in warmer areas of North America, primarily the desert Southwest. Native Americans used yucca's long, swordlike leaves (they look a little like flattened aloe leaves) for fiber, and they used its roots to make soap. In folk medicine, different species have been applied against arthritis, diabetes, bleeding, and sores, among other problems.

Therapeutic Uses:
🍂🍂🍂 Menstrual pain, premenstrual tension.
🍂 Headache, high blood pressure, high cholesterol, high triglycerides, inflammation, intestinal disease, menopause, osteoarthritis, pain, stomach disease, swelling.
▦ Folk uses: Diabetes, gallbladder problems, liver disease, skin cancer.

Medicinal Properties:
Yucca researchers have tested several different species of the plant, so it's difficult to tell precisely which one is responsible for which therapeutic result. What we can say is this: In one clinical study, yucca saponins (the active phytochemicals) alleviated pain, swelling, and stiffness for half of 150 people with arthritis, although relief became apparent anywhere from days to months after the participants began taking the extract. Animal experiments back up the anti-inflammatory action. Another study, involving 212 people, demonstrated a reduction in blood pressure, cholesterol, and triglycerides. Other research indicates that extracts from various yucca species may improve circulation, help digestion, and counteract headaches.

Dosage Options:
One-quarter to ½ cup of fresh roots daily, 1,470 milligrams of a standardized supplement three times a day, or ¼ ounce of dried yucca root in a pint of water three to five times a day.

Safety Rating: 2

Precautions:
None reported, in part because of limited research. However, yucca's use as a food suggests that it probably won't present any problems for most people. Excessive amounts could cause diarrhea. Extremely large doses of saponins can disturb the structural stability of your red blood cells.

Z

ZEDOARY *(Curcuma zedoaria)*

What It Is:

In India, there exists a well-known, widely used demulcent for inflamed mucous membranes, especially for infants and convalescents. It's made from zedoary, a member of the ginger family that resembles its herbal kin (cardamom, ginger, and turmeric) physically, chemically, culinarily, and medicinally. Native to the Himalayas but widely cultivated in India, Sri Lanka, and China, the plant grows only a foot or two tall, often with brown veins coursing across its green leaves. The root is grayish or dirty white. In France, zedoary is known as *zedoaire,* in Germany *zitwer,* and in Spain *cedoaria* or *cetoal.* Indonesians call it *temu putich,* while Malaysians refer to it as *temu kuning.*

Therapeutic Uses:

❧ Alzheimer's disease, arthritis, cancer, colds, gas.

▣ Folk uses: Colic, cramps, indigestion, jaundice, neuroses.

Medicinal Properties:

Think of zedoary as a far weaker version of turmeric (see "Turmeric" on page 215). Like its more famous relative, it contains the phytochemical curcumin, but in a lower concentration (only about 0.1 percent), making turmeric the preferred herbal medicine. Curcumin is an excellent anti-inflammatory for arthritis pain. It also benefits the liver and gallbladder and protects against cancer and Alzheimer's disease. In Asia, zedoary's curcumol and curdione are considered good cancer fighters, especially against cervical cancer and lymphosarcoma.

Curcumin soothes inflamed tissue in much the same way as the relatively new class of nonsteroidal anti-inflammatory drugs (NSAIDs) called cyclooxygenase-2 (COX-2) inhibitors (see "Turmeric" on page 215). It deters the body's release of COX-2 prostaglandins, which are secreted in response to inflammation and swelling. Unlike aspirin, it doesn't tamper with the body's release of related COX-1 prostaglandins, which are necessary for blood clotting and other physiologic functions. (Aspirin prevents the release of both COX-1 and COX-2, which is why it helps against arthritis and thins the blood but also promotes ulcers and increases the chances of intestinal bleeding.)

Prescription Counterparts:
Because zedoary's curcumin concentration is low, don't count on it for much anti-inflammatory help. It does, however, make a nice tag team partner for turmeric. See the prescription counterparts under "Turmeric" on page 216 to learn how well it stacks up against its pharmaceutical rivals.

Dosage Options:
Steep 1 to 1½ teaspoons of dried root in a cup of water and drink as a tea up to three times a day.

Safety Rating: 3

Precautions:
Zedoary is a food, so there's little cause for concern with rational use. Women who experience a heavy menstrual flow should avoid taking large dosages. Extremely large amounts of curcuminoids—more than you're likely able to ingest—might cause ulcers or cancer or might reduce the number of red and white corpuscles in the blood.

PART THREE

GUIDE TO CONDITIONS

If you would like to know what herbs are recommended for a specific health problem, you can use this guide to find the information you need. Simply look up the ailment and turn to the page number or numbers listed to learn more about the herbs that can prevent or treat it.

A

ABDOMINAL CRAMPS
Anise, 29–30
Ashwaganda, 31–32
Basil, 33–34
Black cohosh, 40–41
Boldo, 48
Butcher's broom, 57–58
Caraway, 60–61
Cardamom, 61–62
Catnip, 64–65
Cayenne, 66–68
Chamomile, German, 69–71
Chasteberry, 72–73
Echinacea, 90–92
Eucalyptus, 95–96
Fennel, 100
Feverfew, 102–4
Ginger, 110–12
Goldenseal, 117–18
Hops, 126–27
Juniper, 134
Kava-kava, 135–36
Licorice, 140–43
Meadowsweet, 148–49
Mortherwort, 152
Mullein, 153–54
Passionflower, 166–67
Peppermint, 168–70
Prickly ash, 177–78
Psyllium, 178–79
Raspberry, 181–82
Red clover, 182–84
Rue, 189
Sage, 190–91
St. John's wort, 191–93
Skunk cabbage, 202–3
Spearmint, 205–6
Thyme, 213–14
Valerian, 217–18
Vervain, 219
Yerba santa, 230–31
Zedoary, 234–35

ABDOMINAL DISTRESS (SEE GASTRIC PROBLEMS; STOMACH PROBLEMS)

ABRASIONS
Aloe, 28
Calendula, 58–59
Myrrh, 155
Witch hazel, 224–25

ABSCESSES
Broom, 52–53
Chickweed, 73
Echinacea, 90–92
Fo-ti, 105
Garlic, 106–9
Marshmallow, 146–47
Mistletoe, 151–52
Papaya, 163–64
Slippery elm, 203–4
Sweet Annie, 209–10
Yerba mansa, 229–30

ACETAMINOPHEN POISONING
Garlic, 106–9

ACNE
Aloe, 28
Basil, 33–34
Burdock, 56
Calendula, 58–59
Chamomile, German, 69–71
Chaparral, 71
Chasteberry, 72–73
Echinacea, 90–92
Eucalyptus, 95–96
Goldenseal, 117–18
Gugul, 122–23
Hawthorn, 125–26
Horse chestnut, 127–28
Meadowsweet, 148–49
Onion, 161
Oregon grape, 162
Sage, 190–91
Sassafras, 194–95
Tea tree, 212–13
Valerian, 217–18
Yellow dock, 228–29

ADDICTION, GENERAL (SEE ALSO ALCOHOLISM; DRUG ADDICTION; NICOTINE ADDICTION)
Oats, 159–60
Passionflower, 166–67
Skullcap, 201–2

ADDISON'S DISEASE
Licorice, 140–43

ADENOMA
Pumpkin, 179–80

AGGRESSION
Rhubarb, 185–86

AGING
Ginger, 110–12

AGUE
Nettle, 157–58

ALCOHOLISM
Alfalfa, 27–28
Basil, 33–34
Cayenne, 66–68
Chaparral, 71
Dandelion, 86–87
Evening primrose, 96–97
Ginger, 110–12
Ginseng, Oriental, 115–16
Goldenseal, 117–18
Kudzu, 136–37
St. John's wort, 191–93
Skullcap, 201–2

ALLERGIES (SEE ALSO HAY FEVER)
Cat's claw, 65–66
Chamomile, German, 69–71
Devil's claw, 87
Dong quai, 88–89
Echinacea, 90–92
Ephedra; Ma huang, 94–95
Fenugreek, 101–2
Feverfew, 102–4
Fo-ti, 105
Ginkgo, 112–14
Horseradish, 129
Hydrangea, 131
Kudzu, 136–37

ALLERGIES (cont.)
Nettle, 157–58
Picrorrhiza, 172–73
Yerba santa, 230–31
ALTITUDE SICKNESS
Ginkgo, 112–14
ALVEOLITIS
Dong quai, 88–89
ALZHEIMER'S DISEASE
Ashwaganda, 31–32
Evening primrose, 96–97
Garlic, 106–9
Ginkgo, 112–14
Ginseng, Oriental, 115–16
Lemon balm, 139–40
Lobelia, 144
Rosemary, 187–88
Sage, 190–91
Tea, 210–11
Thyme, 213–14
Turmeric, 215–16
Zedoary, 234–35
AMNESIA
Ginseng, Oriental, 115–16
AMOEBA INFECTIONS
Ipecac, 133
ANAL INFLAMMATION
Horse chestnut, 127–28
ANAPHYLACTIC SHOCK
Grape; Grape seed, 120–21
ANEMIA
Aloe, 28
Anise, 29–30
Artichoke, 30–31
Ashwaganda, 31–32
Caraway, 60–61
Dong quai, 88–89
Fo-ti, 105
Gotu kola, 119–20
Hawthorn, 125–26
Nettle, 157–58
Pau d'arco, 167–68
Rehmannia; Chinese
foxglove, 184–85
Vervain, 219
Wormwood, 226–27
Yellow dock, 228–29
ANGINA
Astragalus, 32–33
ANKYLOSING SPONDYLITIS
White willow, 221–22
ANOREXIA
Burdock, 56

ANXIETY (*SEE ALSO* PANIC)
Blue cohosh, 47
Bugle, 55
Celery seed, 68–69
Chamomile, German, 69–71
Damiana, 85
Evening primrose, 96–97
Ginkgo, 112–14
Ginseng, Oriental, 115–16
Hops, 126–27
Kava-kava, 135–36
Lemon balm, 139–40
Linden, 143
Mistletoe, 151–52
Motherwort, 152
Oats, 159–60
Passionflower, 166–67
St. John's wort, 191–93
Skullcap, 201–2
Valerian, 217–18
Wild cherry, 222–23
Wood betony, 225–26
AORTIC INFLAMMATION
Dong quai, 88–89
APPENDICITIS
Garlic, 106–9
Licorice, 140–43
Rhubarb, 185–86
**APPETITE, LACK OF OR
POOR**
Artichoke, 30–31
Astragalus, 32–33
Blessed thistle, 44–45
Boldo, 48
Boneset, 49
Caraway, 60–61
Cardamom, 61–62
Cayenne, 66–68
Celery seed, 68–69
Chicory, 74–75
Cinnamon and Cassia,
75–76
Cola, 79
Dandelion, 86–87
Devil's claw, 87
Eucalyptus, 95–96
False unicorn root, 99
Fennel, 100
Fenugreek, 101–2
Gentian, 109–10
Ginger, 110–12
Ginseng, Oriental, 115–16
Goldenseal, 117–18

Hops, 126–27
Horseradish, 129
Juniper, 134
Kava-kava, 135–36
Lavender, 138
Licorice, 140–43
Maté, 147
Milk thistle, 149–50
Muira puama, 153
Onion, 161
Papaya, 163–64
Peppermint, 168–70
Picrorrhiza, 172–73
Pineapple, 173–75
Rosemary, 187–88
Sage, 190–91
St. John's wort, 191–93
Soybean, 204–5
Thyme, 213–14
Tomato, 214
Turmeric, 215–16
White horehound, 220
Wild cherry, 222–23
Wormwood, 226–27
Yarrow, 227–28
Yerba mansa, 229–30
ARSENIC POISONING
Artichoke, 30–31
ARTERIAL BLOCKAGES
Gugul, 122–123
**ARTHRITIS (*SEE ALSO*
OSTEOARTHRITIS;
RHEUMATISM;
RHEUMATOID ARTHRITIS)**
Alfalfa, 27–28
Aloe, 28
Artichoke, 30–31
Ashwaganda, 31–32
Basil, 33–34
Bilberry, 37
Birch, 38
Black currant, 41–42
Blessed thistle, 44–45
Bloodroot, 45–46
Blue cohosh, 47
Boneset, 49
Borage, 50
Boswellia, 51
Burdock, 56
Butcher's broom, 57–58
Camphor, 59–60
Cascara sagrada, 63–64
Cat's claw, 65–66

AUTOIMMUNE DISORDERS
Astragalus, 32–33
Black currant, 41–42
Boldo, 48
Picrorrhiza, 172–73
Rehmannia; Chinese
foxglove, 184–85

B

**BACKACHE (SEE ALSO
LUMBAGO; SCIATICA)**
Ashwaganda, 31–32
Burdock, 56
Cayenne, 66–68
Devil's claw, 87
Fo-ti, 105
Ginger, 110–12
Horse chestnut, 127–28
Rehmannia; Chinese
foxglove, 184–85
Yarrow, 227–28
BACTERIAL INFECTIONS
Blessed thistle, 44–45
Camphor, 59–60
Caraway, 60–61
Carob, 62–63
Chicory, 74–75
Olive leaf, 160
Phyllanthus, 171–72
BAD BREATH
Alfalfa, 27–28
Anise, 29–30
Bloodroot, 45–46
Cardamom, 61–62
Clove, 77
Eucalyptus, 95–96
Meadowsweet, 148–49
Parsley, 164–65
Thyme, 213–14
BALDNESS
Birch, 38
Burdock, 56
Evening primrose, 96–97
Fenugreek, 101–2
Garlic, 106–9
Ginger, 110–12
Ginkgo, 112–14
Gotu kola, 119–20
Horsetail, 130
Nettle, 157–58
Parsley, 164–65

Rosemary, 187–88
Saw palmetto, 195–97
Thyme, 213–14
BEDBUGS
Black walnut, 43–44
BEDSORES
Aloe, 28
Chamomile, German, 69–71
Comfrey, 82–83
Garlic, 106–9
Gotu kola, 119–20
Myrrh, 155
BED–WETTING
Bearberry, 35
Corn silk, 83
Damiana, 85
Ephedra; Ma huang, 94–95
Fennel, 100
Horsetail, 130
Kava-kava, 135–36
Nettle, 157–58
Pumpkin, 179–80
Pygeum, 180–81
St. John's wort, 191–93
Thyme, 213–14
BEE STINGS
Calendula, 58–59
BELCHING
Juniper, 134
BILE BLOCKAGE
Peppermint, 168–70
BILIARY SPASMS
Belladonna, 36
**BITES (SEE BUG BITES;
SNAKEBITE)**
BLACK–AND–BLUE MARKS
Parsley, 164–65
BLADDER PROBLEMS
Cranberry, 84
Juniper, 134
Pumpkin, 179–80
Stoneroot, 207
BLADDER STONES
Birch, 38
Black currant, 41–42
Burdock, 56
Corn silk, 83
Dandelion, 86–87
Goldenrod, 116–17
Horsetail, 130
Hydrangea, 131
Maté, 147
Nettle, 157–58

Parsley, 164–65
Pumpkin, 179–80
Stoneroot, 207
Wood betony, 225–26
**BLEEDING, GENERAL (SEE
ALSO HEMORRHAGE;
NOSEBLEEDS)**
Vervain, 219
BLEPHARITIS
Eyebright, 98
BLINDNESS
Aloe, 28
BLOATING
Chamomile, German, 69–71
White horehound, 220
BLOOD CLOTTING
Artichoke, 30–31
Butcher's broom, 57–58
Ginger, 110–12
Ginkgo, 112–14
Horse chestnut, 127–28
Papaya, 163–64
Pineapple, 173–75
Skullcap, 201–2
**BLOOD FLOW DEFICIENCY
TO THE BRAIN**
Ginkgo, 112–14
BLOOD POISONING
Echinacea, 90–92
**BLOOD PRESSURE (SEE
HIGH BLOOD PRESSURE;
LOW BLOOD PRESSURE)**
**BLOOD SUGAR LEVELS
(SEE HIGH BLOOD
SUGAR; LOW BLOOD
SUGAR)**
BOILS
Bitter melon, 38–39
Boswellia, 51
Burdock, 56
Burnet, 57
Chickweed, 73
Devil's claw, 87
Echinacea, 90–92
Elder, European;
Elderberry, 92–93
Fenugreek, 101–2
Flax, 104–5
Gotu kola, 119–20
Hops, 126–27
Licorice, 140–43
Lobelia, 144
Myrrh, 155

Onion, 161
Passionflower, 166–67
Psyllium, 196–97
Slippery elm, 203–4
Sweet Annie, 209–10
Tea tree, 212–13
Tomato, 214
Turmeric, 215–16
BOWEL CRAMPS
Chaparral, 71
BREAST CANCER
Kudzu, 136–37
Milk thistle, 149–50
Plantain, 175–76
BREAST INFLAMMATION
Black cohosh, 40–41
Kudzu, 136–37
Sassafras, 194–95
BREAST MILK DEFICIENCY
Anise, 29–30
Caraway, 60–61
Chasteberry, 72–73
Fennel, 100
Fenugreek, 101–2
Milk thistle, 149–50
Parsley, 164–65
Partridgeberry, 165–66
Vervain, 219
BREAST MILK EXCESS
Sage, 190–91
**BREAST PAIN AND
TENDERNESS**
Bugle, 55
Calendula, 58–59
Chamomile, German,
69–71
Chasteberry, 72–73
Comfrey, 82–83
Dandelion, 86–87
Echinacea, 90–92
Evening primrose, 96–97
Parsley, 164–65
BREATHING PROBLEMS (*SEE*
RESPIRATORY PROBLEMS;
SPECIFIC TYPES)
BRONCHIAL PROBLEMS
Belladonna, 36
Black cohosh, 40–41
Borage, 50
Ephedra; Ma huang, 94–95
Garlic, 106–9
Myrrh, 155
Yellow dock, 228–29

BRONCHIECTASIS
Garlic, 106–9
BRONCHITIS
Aloe, 28
Anise, 29–30
Ashwaganda, 31–32
Bearberry, 35
Black cohosh, 40–41
Bloodroot, 45–46
Boneset, 49
Camphor, 59–60
Caraway, 60–61
Cardamom, 61–62
Catnip, 64–65
Chaparral, 71
Cinnamon and Cassia,
75–76
Clove, 77
Coffee, 78–79
Coltsfoot, 81–82
Comfrey, 82–83
Dandelion, 86–87
Echinacea, 90–92
Elder, European;
Elderberry, 92–93
Elecampane, 93–94
Ephedra; Ma huang, 94–95
Eucalyptus, 95–96
Fennel, 100
Fenugreek, 101–2
Flax, 104–5
Fo-ti, 105
Garlic, 106–9
Gentian, 109–10
Ginkgo, 112–14
Goldenseal, 117–18
Gotu kola, 119–20
Horseradish, 129
Hydrangea, 131
Hyssop, 131–32
Ipecac, 133
Juniper, 134
Kava-kava, 135–36
Lemon balm, 139–40
Licorice, 140–43
Linden, 143
Lobelia, 144
Marshmallow, 146–47
Meadowsweet, 148–49
Mullein, 153–54
Nettle, 157–58
Onion, 161
Papaya, 163–64

Parsley, 164–65
Peppermint, 168–70
Plantain, 175–76
Pleurisy root, 176–77
Red clover, 182–84
Saw palmetto, 195–97
Skunk cabbage, 202–3
Sundew, 208–9
Thyme, 213–14
White horehound, 220
Wild cherry, 222–23
Wood betony, 225–26
Yerba mansa, 229–30
Yerba santa, 230–31
BRONCHOSIS
Birch, 38
BRUISES
Aloe, 28
Basil, 33–34
Bilberry, 37
Buchu, 53–54
Burdock, 56
Chamomile, German, 69–71
Comfrey, 82–83
Dong quai, 88–89
Elder, European;
Elderberry, 92–93
Evening primrose, 96–97
Gotu kola, 119–20
Hops, 126–27
Horse chestnut, 127–28
Lobelia, 144
Marshmallow, 146–47
Meadowsweet, 148–49
Onion, 161
Oregon grape, 162
Parsley, 164–65
Passionflower, 166–67
Pineapple, 173–75
Pleurisy root, 176–77
Rosemary, 187–88
St. John's wort, 191–93
Stoneroot, 207
Tea tree, 212–13
Thyme, 213–14
Turmeric, 215–16
Vervain, 219
Witch hazel, 224–25
Yellow dock, 228–29
Yerba santa, 230–31
BUERGER'S DISEASE
Dong quai, 88–89
Hawthorn, 125–26

BUG BITES
Aloe, 28
Basil, 33–34
Chamomile, German,
69–71
Chickweed, 73
Clove, 77
Comfrey, 82–83
Echinacea, 90–92
Lemon balm, 139–40
Lobelia, 144
Nettle, 157–58
Onion, 161
Peppermint, 168–70
Sage, 190–91
Tea tree, 212–13
Witch hazel, 224–25
Wormwood, 226–27
BUNIONS
Calendula, 58–59
Chamomile, German, 69–71
Clove, 77
Sundew, 208–9
Tea tree, 212–13
Turmeric, 215–16
BURNS
Aloe, 28
Burdock, 56
Burnet, 57
Calendula, 58–59
Camphor, 59–60
Chamomile, German, 69–71
Chaparral, 71
Cleavers, 76
Echinacea, 90–92
Flax, 104–5
Garlic, 106–9
Ginger, 110–12
Gotu kola, 119–20
Horsetail, 130
Hydrangea, 131
Marshmallow, 146–47
Nettle, 157–58
Onion, 161
Papaya, 163–64
Rhubarb, 185–86
St. John's wort, 191–93
Shepherd's purse, 200–1
Slippery elm, 203–4
Stoneroot, 207
Tea tree, 212–13
Tomato, 214
Witch hazel, 224–25

Yarrow, 227–28
Yellow dock, 228–29
BURSITIS
Blessed thistle, 44–45
Boswellia, 51
Cayenne, 66–68
Turmeric, 215–16
White willow, 221–22

C

CALCULUS
Stoneroot, 207
CALLUSES
Tea tree, 212–13
CANCER, GENERAL (SEE ALSO SPECIFIC TYPES)
Alfalfa, 27–28
Ashwaganda, 31–32
Astragalus, 32–33
Birch, 38
Blessed thistle, 44–45
Bloodroot, 45–46
Boldo, 48
Boneset, 49
Calendula, 58–59
Cascara sagrada, 63–64
Cat's claw, 65–66
Chamomile, German, 69–71
Chicory, 74–75
Cleavers, 76
Devil's claw, 87
Echinacea, 90–92
Evening primrose, 96–97
Fenugreek, 101–2
Flax, 104–5
Garlic, 106–9
Ginseng, Oriental, 115–16
Goldenseal, 117–18
Grape; Grape seed, 120–21
Hydrangea, 131
Juniper, 134
Lavender, 138
Mistletoe, 151–52
Myrrh, 155
Nettle, 157–58
Onion, 161
Pau d'arco, 167–68
Pineapple, 173–75
Prickly ash, 177–78
Red clover, 182–84
Rhubarb, 185–86

Rosemary, 187–88
Sage, 190–91
Sarsaparilla, 193–94
Schisandra, 198
Spearmint, 205–6
Suma, 208
Tea, 210–11
Thyme, 213–14
Tomato, 214
Turmeric, 215–16
White willow, 221–22
Wild cherry, 222–23
Yerba santa, 230–31
Zedoary, 234–35
CANKER SORES
Burdock, 56
Chamomile, German, 69–71
Echinacea, 90–92
Goldenseal, 117–18
Licorice, 140–43
Myrrh, 155
Raspberry, 181–82
Sage, 190–91
CAPILLARY FRAGILITY
Ginkgo, 112–14
Grape; Grape seed, 120–21
Rose hips, 186–87
CARBUNCLES
Ashwaganda, 31–32
Echinacea, 90–92
Rhubarb, 185–86
CARDIAC INSUFFICIENCY
Belladonna, 36
Shepherd's purse, 200–1
CARDIOPATHY (SEE HEART DISEASE)
CARDIOVASCULAR PROBLEMS
Bilberry, 37
Hawthorn, 125–26
CARIES
Grape; Grape seed, 120–21
Licorice, 140–43
CARPAL TUNNEL SYNDROME
Horse chestnut, 127–28
CATARACTS
Bilberry, 37
Catnip, 64–65
Ginger, 110–12
Licorice, 140–43
Rehmannia; Chinese
foxglove, 184–85

CYTOMEGALOVIRUS
Garlic, 106–9
St. John's wort, 191–93

D

DANDRUFF
Birch, 38
Echinacea, 90–92
Ginger, 110–12
Goldenseal, 117–18
Myrrh, 155
Oregon grape, 162
Plantain, 175–76
Soybean, 204–5
Tea tree, 212–13
DEAFNESS
Ginkgo, 112–14
Kudzu, 136–37
DEBILITY
Kava-kava, 135–36
Oats, 159–60
Periwinkle, 170–71
Saw palmetto, 195–97
Vervain, 219
Wild cherry, 222–23
DELIRIUM
Rhubarb, 185–86
DEMENTIA
Chasteberry, 72–73
Evening primrose, 96–97
Gotu kola, 119–20
Lavender, 138
DENGUE
Boneset, 49
DENTAL PROBLEMS (SEE
ALSO **CAVITIES; GUM
DISEASE; TOOTHACHE)**
Basil, 33–34
Chamomile, German, 69–71
Echinacea, 90–92
Horseradish, 129
Tea, 210–11
Thyme, 213–14
DEPRESSION (SEE ALSO
MELANCHOLY)
Basil, 33–34
Borage, 50
Celery seed, 68–69
Chasteberry, 72–73
Cola, 79
Damiana, 85

Ginger, 110–12
Ginkgo, 112–14
Ginseng, Oriental, 115–16
Hops, 126–27
Lavender, 138
Licorice, 140–43
Maté, 147
Oats, 159–60
Papaya, 163–64
Passionflower, 166–67
Sage, 190–91
St. John's wort, 191–93
Schisandra, 198
Spearmint, 205–6
Thyme, 213–14
Valerian, 217–18
Vervain, 219
Yohimbe, 231–32
DERMATITIS
Aloe, 28
Ashwaganda, 31–32
Bayberry, 34
Bilberry, 37
Boneset, 49
Borage, 50
Burdock, 56
Burnet, 57
Calendula, 58–59
Chickweed, 73
Chicory, 74–75
Cleavers, 76
Clove, 77
Elecampane, 93–94
Evening primrose, 96–97
Fenugreek, 101–2
Feverfew, 102–4
Flax, 104–5
Fo-ti, 105
Ginkgo, 112–14
Goldenseal, 117–18
Marshmallow, 146–47
Milk thistle, 149–50
Mullein, 153–54
Myrrh, 155
Neem, 156
Nettle, 157–58
Oats, 159–60
Oregon grape, 162
Pau d'arco, 167–68
Psyllium, 196–97
Red clover, 182–84
Rehmannia; Chinese
foxglove, 184–85

Sage, 190–91
St. John's wort, 191–93
Sarsaparilla, 193–94
Sassafras, 194–95
Senna, 199–200
Slippery elm, 203–4
Tea tree, 212–13
Thyme, 213–14
Turmeric, 215–16
Witch hazel, 224–25
Wood betony, 225–26
Yellow dock, 228–29
Yerba santa, 230–31
DIABETES
Alfalfa, 27–28
Aloe, 28
Astragalus, 32–33
Bearberry, 35
Bilberry, 37
Bitter melon, 38–39
Bugle, 55
Cayenne, 66–68
Celery seed, 68–69
Damiana, 85
Dandelion, 86–87
Echinacea, 90–92
Elecampane, 93–94
Eucalyptus, 95–96
Evening primrose, 96–97
Fenugreek, 101–2
Fo-ti, 105
Garlic, 106–9
Ginkgo, 112–14
Ginseng, Oriental, 115–16
Goldenrod, 116–17
Goldenseal, 117–18
Gymnema, 123–24
Juniper, 134
Kudzu, 136–37
Lavender, 138
Licorice, 140–43
Marshmallow, 146–47
Milk thistle, 149–50
Myrrh, 155
Neem, 156
Oats, 159–60
Olive leaf, 160
Onion, 161
Phyllanthus, 171–72
Psyllium, 196–97
Raspberry, 181–82
Rehmannia; Chinese
foxglove, 184–85

FROSTBITE
Aloe, 28
Calendula, 58–59
Cayenne, 66–68
Chamomile, German, 69–71
Horsetail, 130
Oats, 159–60
FROSTBITE PREVENTION
Hyssop, 131–32
FUNGAL DISEASE AND INFECTIONS
Black walnut, 43–44
Bloodroot, 45–46
Garlic, 106–9
Olive leaf, 160
Pau d'arco, 167–68
Tea tree, 212–13
Thyme, 213–14

G

GALLBLADDER PROBLEMS
Anise, 29–30
Artichoke, 30–31
Belladonna, 36
Caraway, 60–61
Cardamom, 61–62
Chamomile, German, 69–71
Chicory, 74–75
Dandelion, 86–87
Devil's claw, 87
Echinacea, 90–92
Eucalyptus, 95–96
Flax, 104–5
Goldenseal, 117–18
Horseradish, 129
Horsetail, 130
Hydrangea, 131
Hyssop, 131–32
Kava-kava, 135–36
Lavender, 138
Licorice, 140–43
Linden, 143
Marshmallow, 146–47
Milk thistle, 149–50
Nettle, 157–58
Oats, 159–60
Papaya, 163–64
Peppermint, 168–70
Rhubarb, 185–86
Rosemary, 187–88
St. John's wort, 191–93

Saw palmetto, 195–97
Turmeric, 215–16
White horehound, 220
Wood betony, 225–26
Wormwood, 226–27
Yarrow, 227–28
Yucca, 233
GALLSTONES
Artichoke, 30–31
Boldo, 48
Broom, 52–53
Cascara sagrada, 63–64
Celery seed, 68–69
Dandelion, 86–87
Milk thistle, 149–50
Parsley, 164–65
Turmeric, 215–16
Wild yam, 223–24
GANGRENE
Blessed thistle, 44–45
GAS
Anise, 29–30
Artichoke, 30–31
Basil, 33–34
Calendula, 58–59
Caraway, 60–61
Cardamom, 61–62
Cascara sagrada, 63–64
Catnip, 64–65
Cayenne, 66–68
Celery seed, 68–69
Chamomile, German, 69–71
Cinnamon and Cassia, 75–76
Dandelion, 86–87
Elecampane, 93–94
Fennel, 100
Fenugreek, 101–2
Garlic, 106–9
Gentian, 109–10
Ginger, 110–12
Hyssop, 131–32
Juniper, 134
Lavender, 138
Lemon balm, 139–40
Motherwort, 152
Myrrh, 155
Papaya, 163–64
Peppermint, 168–70
Pineapple, 173–75
Rhubarb, 185–86
Rosemary, 187–88
Spearmint, 205–6

Sweet Annie, 209–10
Thyme, 213–14
Turmeric, 215–16
White horehound, 220
Wormwood, 226–27
Zedoary, 234–35
GASTRIC PROBLEMS
Bilberry, 37
Echinacea, 90–92
Elecampane, 93–94
Evening primrose, 96–97
Fennel, 100
Gentian, 109–10
Lemon balm, 139–40
Rhubarb, 185–86
Rosemary, 187–88
Spearmint, 205–6
GASTRIC REFLUX
Meadowsweet, 148–49
GASTRITIS
Bayberry, 34
Blackberry, 40
Calendula, 58–59
Cat's claw, 65–66
Chamomile, German, 69–71
Comfrey, 82–83
Dandelion, 86–87
Fenugreek, 101–2
Flax, 104–5
Gentian, 109–10
Ginger, 110–12
Ginseng, Oriental, 115–16
Goldenseal, 117–18
Kudzu, 136–37
Marshmallow, 146–47
Passionflower, 166–67
Peppermint, 168–70
Rose hips, 186–87
Slippery elm, 203–4
Sundew, 208–9
Thyme, 213–14
Wild yam, 223–24
Wormwood, 226–27
Yarrow, 227–28
GASTRODUODENITIS
St. John's wort, 191–93
GASTROENTERITIS
Garlic, 106–9
GINGIVITIS
Bayberry, 34
Bloodroot, 45–46
Goldenseal, 117–18
Myrrh, 155

Neem, 156
Peppermint, 168–70
Rhubarb, 185–86
Sage, 190–91
Thyme, 213–14
Witch hazel, 224–25
Wood betony, 225–26
Yellow dock, 228–29
Yerba mansa, 229–30

GLANDS, SWOLLEN
Fenugreek, 101–2

GLAUCOMA
Aloe, 28
Bilberry, 37
Catnip, 64–65
Coleus Forskohlii, 80–81

GOITER
Echinacea, 90–92
Nettle, 157–58

GONORRHEA
Bearberry, 35
Boldo, 48
Corn silk, 83
Echinacea, 90–92
Goldenseal, 117–18
Horsetail, 130
Kava-kava, 135–36
Phyllanthus, 171–72
Sarsaparilla, 193–94
Senna, 199–200
Yerba mansa, 229–30

GOUT
Artichoke, 30–31
Bilberry, 37
Birch, 38
Blackberry, 40
Black currant, 41–42
Boldo, 48
Boneset, 49
Broom, 52–53
Burdock, 56
Cat's claw, 65–66
Celery seed, 68–69
Chamomile, German, 69–71
Chickweed, 73
Chicory, 74–75
Corn silk, 83
Cranberry, 84
Dandelion, 86–87
Devil's claw, 87
Fenugreek, 101–2
Flax, 104–5
Goldenrod, 116–17

Grape; Grape seed, 120–21
Horseradish, 129
Horsetail, 130
Hyssop, 131–32
Juniper, 134
Kava-kava, 135–36
Meadowsweet, 148–49
Mistletoe, 151–52
Nettle, 157–58
Oats, 159–60
Olive leaf, 160
Psyllium, 196–97
Rose hips, 186–87
Sassafras, 194–95
Vervain, 219
White willow, 221–22
Wood betony, 225–26
Wormwood, 226–27

GRAVEL
Horsetail, 130
Hydrangea, 131
Meadowsweet, 148–49
Nettle, 157–58
Parsley, 164–65

GRAVES' DISEASE (SEE
THYROID DISEASE)

GRAYING HAIR
Fo-ti, 105
Rehmannia; Chinese
foxglove, 184–85

**GUM DISEASE AND
PROBLEMS (**SEE ALSO
**GINGIVITIS;
PERIODONTITIS)**
Bilberry, 37
Burnet, 57
Chamomile, German, 69–71
Clove, 77
Comfrey, 82–83
Echinacea, 90–92
Eucalyptus, 95–96
Garlic, 106–9
Goldenseal, 117–18
Gugul, 122–123
Myrrh, 155
Neem, 156
Peppermint, 168–70
Rhubarb, 185–86
Sage, 190–91
Tea, 210–11
Thyme, 213–14
Valerian, 217–18
Witch hazel, 224–25

Wood betony, 225–26
Yellow dock, 228–29
Yerba mansa, 229–30

H

HAIR LOSS (SEE **BALDNESS)**
HALITOSIS (SEE **BAD
BREATH)**
HANGOVER
Kudzu, 136–37
Tomato, 214
**HARDENING OF THE
ARTERIES**
Bilberry, 37
Boldo, 48
Buckwheat, 54
Cayenne, 66–68
Corn silk, 83
Dong quai, 88–89
Evening primrose, 96–97
Fenugreek, 101–2
Fo-ti, 105
Garlic, 106–9
Ginger, 110–12
Ginkgo, 112–14
Grape; Grape seed, 120–21
Gugul, 122–123
Hawthorn, 125–26
Linden, 143
Mistletoe, 151–52
Oats, 159–60
Onion, 161
Papaya, 163–64
Psyllium, 196–97
Rosemary, 187–88
Sundew, 208–9
Turmeric, 215–16
HAY FEVER
Alfalfa, 27–28
Ephedra; Ma huang, 94–95
Fenugreek, 101–2
Nettle, 157–58
Yerba santa, 230–31
HEADACHE
Black haw, 42–43
Cayenne, 66–68
Chasteberry, 72–73
Coffee, 78–79
Cola, 79
Damiana, 85
Devil's claw, 87

KIDNEY STONES (cont.)
Pineapple, 173–75
Stoneroot, 207
Wood betony, 225–26
Wormwood, 226–27
KNEE PAIN
Fo-ti, 105

L

LABOR
False unicorn root, 99
Fenugreek, 101–2
Ginkgo, 112–14
Lavender, 138
Meadowsweet, 148–49
Motherwort, 152
Nettle, 157–58
Parsley, 164–65
Partridgeberry, 165–66
Pineapple, 173–75
Raspberry, 181–82
Schisandra, 198
Shepherd's purse, 200–1
Wild cherry, 222–23
Wild yam, 223–24
LABOR INDUCTION
Blue cohosh, 47
LARYNGITIS
Cayenne, 66–68
Elder, European;
Elderberry, 92–93
Garlic, 106–9
Goldenseal, 117–18
Lobelia, 144
Sage, 190–91
Stoneroot, 207
Sundew, 208–9
Thyme, 213–14
White horehound, 220
Yerba mansa, 229–30
LEAD POISONING
Garlic, 106–9
LEG CRAMPS
Horse chestnut, 127–28
LEISHMANIASIS
Picrorrhiza, 172–73
Sundew, 208–9
Sweet Annie, 209–10
LEPROSY
Bitter melon, 38–39
Gotu kola, 119–20

Hops, 126–27
Kava-kava, 135–36
Myrrh, 155
Sarsaparilla, 193–94
LETHARGY
Cola, 79
Ephedra; Ma huang, 94–95
Rosemary, 187–88
LEUKEMIA
Cascara sagrada, 63–64
Kudzu, 136–37
Papaya, 163–64
Pau d'arco, 167–68
LEUKOCYTOSIS
Ashwaganda, 31–32
LEUKOPENIA (*SEE* WHITE BLOOD CELL COUNT, LOW)
LIBIDO, LOW
Anise, 29–30
Artichoke, 30–31
Ashwaganda, 31–32
Damiana, 85
Dong quai, 88–89
Fennel, 100
Fenugreek, 101–2
Ginger, 110–12
Ginseng, Oriental, 115–16
Gugul, 122–123
Muira puama, 153
Parsley, 164–65
Saw palmetto, 195–97
Yohimbe, 231–32
LICE
Bitter melon, 38–39
Parsley, 164–65
Tea tree, 212–13
Thyme, 213–14
LICHEN PLANUS
Licorice, 140–43
LITHURIA
Stoneroot, 207
LIVER CANCER
Echinacea, 90–92
Ginseng, Oriental, 115–16
LIVER DISEASE AND PROBLEMS
Aloes, 29
Anise, 29–30
Artichoke, 30–31
Belladonna, 36
Black currant, 41–42
Blessed thistle, 44–45

Boldo, 48
Broom, 52–53
Burdock, 56
Calendula, 58–59
Caraway, 60–61
Cardamom, 61–62
Cascara sagrada, 63–64
Celery seed, 68–69
Chamomile, German, 69–71
Chicory, 74–75
Corn silk, 83
Dandelion, 86–87
Devil's claw, 87
Dong quai, 88–89
Elecampane, 93–94
Eucalyptus, 95–96
Evening primrose, 96–97
False unicorn root, 99
Fennel, 100
Garlic, 106–9
Ginger, 110–12
Ginseng, Oriental, 115–16
Horse chestnut, 127–28
Horseradish, 129
Hyssop, 131–32
Kudzu, 136–37
Meadowsweet, 148–49
Oats, 159–60
Oregon grape, 162
Papaya, 163–64
Parsley, 164–65
Peppermint, 184–86
Rosemary, 187–88
Rue, 189
Sassafras, 194–95
Vervain, 219
White horehound, 220
Wormwood, 226–27
Yarrow, 227–28
Yellow dock, 228–29
Yucca, 233
LOW BLOOD PRESSURE
Belladonna, 36
Broom, 52–53
Ephedra; Ma huang, 94–95
Rhubarb, 185–86
Rosemary, 187–88
LOW BLOOD SUGAR
Bilberry, 37
LUMBAGO
Ashwaganda, 31–32
Black cohosh, 40–41
Cayenne, 66–68

Devil's claw, 87
Ginger, 110–12
Rehmannia; Chinese
foxglove, 184–85
LUNG CANCER
Ashwaganda, 31–32
Ginseng, Oriental, 115–16
**LUNG DISEASE AND
PROBLEMS**
Blue cohosh, 47
Broom, 52–53
Bugle, 55
Cayenne, 66–68
Chickweed, 73
Coffee, 78–79
Coltsfoot, 81–82
Dong quai, 88–89
Flax, 104–5
Hyssop, 131–32
Picrorrhiza, 172–73
Pleurisy root, 176–77
Prickly ash, 177–78
Raspberry, 181–82
Red clover, 182–84
Witch hazel, 224–25
Wood betony, 225–26
LUPUS
Flax, 104–5
Gotu kola, 119–20
Horse chestnut, 127–28
Licorice, 140–43
LYMPH GLAND PROBLEMS
Calendula, 58–59
Cleavers, 76
Coltsfoot, 81–82
Echinacea, 90–92
Fo-ti, 105
Papaya, 163–64
Psyllium, 196–97
Turmeric, 215–16
Yellow dock, 228–29
LYMPHOMA
Burdock, 56
Papaya, 163–64

M

MACULAR DEGENERATION
Bilberry, 37
Clove, 77
Ginkgo, 112–14
Grape; Grape seed, 120–21

MALARIA
Boneset, 49
Cayenne, 66–68
Flax, 104–5
Guarana, 121–22
Horse chestnut, 127–28
Licorice, 140–43
Milk thistle, 149–50
Neem, 156
Pau d'arco, 167–68
Picrorrhiza, 172–73
Sweet Annie, 209–10
Vervain, 219
Wormwood, 226–27
MALE MENOPAUSE
Anise, 29–30
**MAMMARY INFLAMMATION
(SEE BREAST
INFLAMMATION)**
MEASLES
Burdock, 56
Echinacea, 90–92
Eucalyptus, 95–96
Gotu kola, 119–20
Kudzu, 136–37
Rehmannia; Chinese
foxglove, 184–85
Sassafras, 194–95
**MELANCHOLY (SEE ALSO
DEPRESSION)**
Cola, 79
Lemon balm, 139–40
Vervain, 219
MELANOMA
Cat's claw, 65–66
MEMORY PROBLEMS
Gotu kola, 119–20
MÉNIÈRE'S DISEASE
Schisandra, 198
MENINGITIS
Echinacea, 90–92
MENOPAUSE
Alfalfa, 27–28
Black cohosh, 40–41
Borage, 50
Chasteberry, 72–73
Dong quai, 88–89
False unicorn root, 99
Fennel, 100
Ginseng, Oriental, 115–16
Kava-kava, 135–36
Red clover, 182–84
St. John's wort, 191–93

Soybean, 204–5
Suma, 208
Vervain, 219
Wild yam, 223–24
Yucca, 233
**MENSTRUAL PAIN AND
PROBLEMS**
Aloes, 29
Bilberry, 37
Black cohosh, 40–41
Black haw, 42–43
Blessed thistle, 44–45
Blue cohosh, 47
Calendula, 58–59
Caraway, 60–61
Catnip, 64–65
Cayenne, 66–68
Celery seed, 68–69
Chamomile, German, 69–71
Chasteberry, 72–73
Cinnamon and Cassia,
75–76
Damiana, 85
Dong quai, 88–89
Elecampane, 93–94
Evening primrose, 96–97
False unicorn root, 99
Fennel, 100
Feverfew, 102–4
Ginger, 110–12
Ginkgo, 112–14
Goldenseal, 117–18
Gotu kola, 119–20
Guarana, 121–22
Gugul, 122–123
Hops, 126–27
Horse chestnut, 127–28
Hyssop, 131–32
Juniper, 134
Kava-kava, 135–36
Lavender, 138
Lemon balm, 139–40
Licorice, 140–43
Meadowsweet, 148–49
Milk thistle, 149–50
Mistletoe, 151–52
Motherwort, 152
Muira puama, 153
Nettle, 157–58
Oats, 159–60
Onion, 161
Parsley, 164–65
Partridgeberry, 165–66

White willow, 221–22
Wild yam, 223–24
Witch hazel, 224–25
Yerba mansa, 229–30
MUSCLE TONE PROBLEMS
Lemon balm, 139–40
MUSHROOM POISONING
Milk thistle, 149–50
Picrorrhiza, 172–73
MYALGIA
Black cohosh, 40–41
St. John's wort, 191–93
MYASTHENIA GRAVIS
Ephedra; Ma huang, 94–95
**MYOCARDIAL
INFLAMMATION**
Hawthorn, 125–26
MYOCARDITIS
Astragalus, 32–33

N

NAILS, BRITTLE
Horsetail, 130
NAIL INFECTIONS
Thyme, 213–14
**NASAL DISEASE AND
PROBLEMS (**SEE ALSO
CONGESTION**)**
Ginkgo, 112–14
Myrrh, 155
Pleurisy root, 176–77
**NASAL MEMBRANE
DISORDERS**
Eyebright, 98
NASAL POLYPS
Bloodroot, 45–46
NAUSEA
Anise, 29–30
Artichoke, 30–31
Ashwaganda, 31–32
Basil, 33–34
Caraway, 60–61
Elecampane, 93–94
Fennel, 100
Feverfew, 102–4
Garlic, 106–9
Gentian, 109–10
Ginger, 110–12
Lemon balm, 139–40
Milk thistle, 149–50
Peppermint, 168–70

Raspberry, 181–82
Spearmint, 205–6
Tea, 210–11
Valerian, 217–18
NEARSIGHTEDNESS
Bilberry, 37
NERVE INFLAMMATION
Fo-ti, 105
Papaya, 163–64
NERVE PAIN
Cayenne, 66–68
Cinnamon and Cassia,
75–76
Cola, 79
Dong quai, 88–89
Eucalyptus, 95–96
Fenugreek, 101–2
Garlic, 106–9
Ginkgo, 112–14
Ginseng, Oriental, 115–16
Guarana, 121–22
Hops, 126–27
Horse chestnut, 127–28
Juniper, 134
Kava-kava, 135–36
Lemon balm, 139–40
Maté, 147
Nettle, 157–58
Passionflower, 166–67
Peppermint, 168–70
Rosemary, 187–88
St. John's wort, 191–93
Thyme, 213–14
Valerian, 217–18
Wood betony, 225–26
NERVOUS EXHAUSTION
Fo-ti, 105
NERVOUSNESS
Black cohosh, 40–41
Bugle, 55
Camphor, 59–60
Caraway, 60–61
Hops, 126–27
Kava-kava, 135–36
Lavender, 138
Lemon balm, 139–40
Linden, 143
Mistletoe, 151–52
Passionflower, 166–67
St. John's wort, 191–93
Shepherd's purse, 200–1
Valerian, 217–18
Wood betony, 225–26

**NERVOUS SYSTEM
PROBLEMS**
Black cohosh, 40–41
Cleavers, 76
NERVOUS TENSION
Skullcap, 201–2
Valerian, 217–18
NEURALGIA
Black cohosh, 40–41
Motherwort, 152
NEURASTHENIA
Oats, 159–60
Papaya, 163–64
Pineapple, 173–75
Schisandra, 198
Vervain, 219
NEUROPATHY, DIABETIC
Cayenne, 66–68
Evening primrose, 96–97
Milk thistle, 149–50
NEUROSES
Belladonna, 36
Chasteberry, 72–73
Feverfew, 102–4
Ginseng, Oriental, 115–16
Gotu kola, 119–20
Hops, 126–27
Juniper, 134
Mistletoe, 151–52
Motherwort, 152
Peppermint, 168–70
Periwinkle, 170–71
Prickly ash, 177–78
St. John's wort, 191–93
Valerian, 217–18
Vervain, 219
Wood betony, 225–26
Zedoary, 234–35
NICOTINE ADDICTION
Garlic, 106–9
Gentian, 109–10
Lobelia, 144
Oats, 159–60
NIGHT BLINDNESS
Bilberry, 37
Grape; Grape seed, 120–21
NIGHT SWEATS
Sage, 190–91
Sweet Annie, 209–10
NOSEBLEEDS
Gotu kola, 119–20
Horsetail, 130
Nettle, 157–58

PSORIASIS (cont.)
  Evening primrose, 96–97
  Gotu kola, 119–20
  Juniper, 134
  Kudzu, 136–37
  Lavender, 138
  Milk thistle, 149–50
  Oregon grape, 162
  Papaya, 163–64
  Pau d'arco, 167–68
  Picrorrhiza, 172–73
  Plantain, 175–76
  Psyllium, 196–97
  Red clover, 182–84
  Sarsaparilla, 193–94
  Turmeric, 215–16
  Yellow dock, 228–29
PSYCHOSIS
  Schisandra, 198

R

RABIES
  Skullcap, 201–2
RADIATION BURNS AND EXPOSURE
  Aloe, 28
  Chamomile, German, 69–71
  Ginseng, Oriental, 115–16
  St. John's wort, 191–93
RASHES
  Comfrey, 82–83
  Rehmannia; Chinese
    foxglove, 184–85
  Yarrow, 227–28
RAYNAUD'S DISEASE
  Bilberry, 37
  Evening primrose, 96–97
  Garlic, 106–9
  Ginkgo, 112–14
  Prickly ash, 177–78
RECTAL PROBLEMS (SEE ALSO HEMORRHOIDS)
  Chamomile, German, 69–71
  Papaya, 163–64
  Psyllium, 196–97
  Yerba mansa, 229–30
RESPIRATORY PROBLEMS
  Catnip, 64–65
  Chamomile, German, 69–71
  Chickweed, 73
  Coleus Forskohlii, 80–81

Coltsfoot, 81–82
  Dandelion, 86–87
  Echinacea, 90–92
  Elder, European;
    Elderberry, 92–93
  Elecampane, 93–94
  Ephedra; Ma huang, 94–95
  Eucalyptus, 95–96
  Fennel, 100
  Fenugreek, 101–2
  Garlic, 106–9
  Ginseng, Oriental, 115–16
  Hawthorn, 125–26
  Horseradish, 129
  Horsetail, 130
  Licorice, 140–43
  Marshmallow, 146–47
  Mullein, 153–54
  Papaya, 163–64
  Peppermint, 168–70
  Pineapple, 173–75
  St. John's wort, 191–93
  Sassafras, 194–95
  Thyme, 213–14
  White horehound, 220
  Wild cherry, 222–23
  Yerba santa, 230–31
RESTLESSNESS
  Hops, 126–27
  Kava-kava, 135–36
  Lavender, 138
  Lemon balm, 139–40
  Passionflower, 166–67
  Rehmannia; Chinese
    foxglove, 184–85
  Valerian, 217–18
RETINAL DISEASE
  Bilberry, 37
  Ginkgo, 112–14
  Grape; Grape seed, 120–21
  Licorice, 140–43
RHEUMATISM
  Alfalfa, 27–28
  Artichoke, 30–31
  Ashwaganda, 31–32
  Basil, 33–34
  Birch, 38
  Black cohosh, 40–41
  Bloodroot, 45–46
  Blue cohosh, 47
  Boldo, 48
  Broom, 52–53
  Yerba santa, 230–31

RHEUMATOID ARTHRITIS
  Picrorrhiza, 172–73
  White willow, 221–22
  Wild yam, 223–24
RHINITIS
  Horseradish, 129
  Nettle, 157–58
  Sage, 190–91
  Yellow dock, 228–29
  Yerba mansa, 229–30
RIB PAIN
  Rosemary, 187–88
RINGWORM
  Aloe, 28
  Ashwaganda, 31–32
  Basil, 33–34
  Black walnut, 43–44
  Boswellia, 51
  Cascara sagrada, 63–64
  Eucalyptus, 95–96
  Fo-ti, 105
  Garlic, 106–9
  Lobelia, 144
  Papaya, 163–64
  Senna, 199–200
  Tomato, 214
  Turmeric, 215–16
  Yellow dock, 228–29
ROUNDWORM
  Garlic, 106–9
  Pumpkin, 179–80
  Wormwood, 226–27

S

SCABIES
  Anise, 29–30
  Ginkgo, 112–14
  Neem, 156
  Pau d'arco, 167–68
  Turmeric, 215–16
SCARS
  Gotu kola, 119–20
SCARLET FEVER
  Burdock, 56
  Echinacea, 90–92
  Eucalyptus, 95–96
SCHISTOSOMIASIS
  Pau d'arco, 167–68
SCHIZOPHRENIA
  Evening primrose,
    96–97

Fo-ti, 105
Gotu kola, 119–20

SCIATICA
Black cohosh, 40–41
Broom, 52–53
Burdock, 56
Chamomile, German,
69–71
Goldenseal, 117–18
Horseradish, 129
Motherwort, 152
Nettle, 157–58
Rose hips, 186–87
Rosemary, 187–88
St. John's wort, 191–93

SCLERODERMA
Gotu kola, 119–20
Thyme, 213–14

SEASICKNESS
Ginger, 110–12

**SEASONAL AFFECTIVE
DISORDER (SAD),**
St. John's wort, 191–93

SEBORRHEA
Aloe, 28
Aloes, 29
Burdock, 56
Hawthorn, 125–26
Oats, 159–60

**SEMEN DISCHARGE,
INVOLUNTARY AND
WITHOUT ORGASM**
Rehmannia; Chinese
foxglove, 184–85

SENILITY
Blue cohosh, 47
Ginkgo, 112–14
Periwinkle, 170–71
Schisandra, 198

SEPTIC SHOCK
Rosemary, 187–88

SEXUAL DESIRE, LOW
(*SEE* **LIBIDO, LOW**)

SEXUAL DYSFUNCTION
Ginkgo, 112–14

**SEXUAL MATURITY,
RETARDED**
Chasteberry, 72–73

SHELL SHOCK
Valerian, 217–18

SHINGLES
Cascara sagrada, 63–64
Cayenne, 66–68

Lemon balm, 139–40
Rhubarb, 185–86

SHOCK
Ginkgo, 112–14
Ginseng, Oriental, 115–16

**SINUS DISEASE AND
PROBLEMS**
Echinacea, 90–92
Pineapple, 173–75
Yerba mansa, 229–30

SINUSITIS
Elder, European;
Elderberry, 92–93
Ephedra; Ma huang, 94–95
Eucalyptus, 95–96
Eyebright, 98
Horseradish, 129
Myrrh, 155
Peppermint, 168–70

SJÖGREN'S SYNDROME
Evening primrose, 96–97

SKIN CANCER
Birch, 38
Chaparral, 71
Pau d'arco, 167–68
Yucca, 233

SKIN PROBLEMS, GENERAL
(*SEE ALSO SPECIFIC
TYPES*)
Aloe, 28
Birch, 38
Calendula, 58–59
Chamomile, German, 69–71
Coleus Forskohlii, 80–81
Dandelion, 86–87
Devil's claw, 87
Echinacea, 90–92
Eucalyptus, 95–96
Evening primrose, 96–97
Garlic, 106–9
Gotu kola, 119–20
Gymnema, 123–24
Hawthorn, 125–26
Kava-kava, 135–36
Lavender, 138
Myrrh, 155
Nettle, 157–58
Parsley, 164–65
Raspberry, 181–82
Rue, 189
Valerian, 217–18
White horehound, 220
White willow, 221–22

Wormwood, 226–27
Yellow dock, 228–29

SLEEPINESS
Coffee, 78–79
Rosemary, 187–88

SMALLPOX
Burdock, 56
Goldenseal, 117–18
Gotu kola, 119–20

SNAKEBITE
Artichoke, 30–31
Basil, 33–34
Black cohosh, 40–41
Broom, 52–53
Chaparral, 71
Echinacea, 90–92
Fennel, 100
Gymnema, 123–24
Juniper, 134
Licorice, 140–43
Picrorrhiza, 172–73

SORES
Aloe, 28
Ashwaganda, 31–32
Bayberry, 34
Blessed thistle, 44–45
Burdock, 56
Calendula, 58–59
Camphor, 59–60
Chamomile, German, 69–71
Chickweed, 73
Cleavers, 76
Clove, 77
Comfrey, 82–83
Devil's claw, 87
Elder, European;
Elderberry, 92–93
Eucalyptus, 95–96
Fenugreek, 101–2
Fo-ti, 105
Garlic, 106–9
Ginkgo, 112–14
Goldenseal, 117–18
Gotu kola, 119–20
Gugul, 122–123
Horse chestnut, 127–28
Hyssop, 131–32
Juniper, 134
Kudzu, 136–37
Lobelia, 144
Marshmallow, 146–47
Mistletoe, 151–52
Mullein, 153–54

THREADWORM
Wormwood, 226–27
THROAT INFLAMMATION
(*SEE ALSO* **SORE THROAT**)
Fennel, 100
THROMBOPHLEBITIS
Calendula, 58–59
Horse chestnut, 127–28
Pineapple, 173–75
THROMBOSIS
Rehmannia; Chinese
foxglove, 184–85
Skullcap, 201–2
Yarrow, 227–28
THRUSH
Licorice, 140–43
Plantain, 175–76
Yerba santa, 230–31
THUMB SUCKING
Cayenne, 66–68
THYROID DISEASE
Black walnut, 43–44
Bugle, 55
Cayenne, 66–68
Coleus Forskohlii, 80–81
Lemon balm, 139–40
Motherwort, 152
Nettle, 157–58
Rehmannia; Chinese
foxglove, 184–85
TINNITUS
Black cohosh, 40–41
Dong quai, 88–89
Feverfew, 102–4
Fo-ti, 105
Ginkgo, 112–14
Goldenseal, 117–18
Rehmannia; Chinese
foxglove, 184–85
TISSUE SWELLING
(*SEE* **SWELLING**)
TOBACCO ADDICTION (*SEE*
NICOTINE ADDICTION)
TONGUE INFLAMMATION
Rehmannia; Chinese
foxglove, 184–85
Rhubarb, 185–86
Sage, 190–91
TONSILLITIS
Coltsfoot, 81–82
Dandelion, 86–87
Echinacea, 90–92
Myrrh, 155

Periwinkle, 170–71
Prickly ash, 177–78
Raspberry, 181–82
Sage, 190–91
Thyme, 213–14
TOOTHACHE
Calendula, 58–59
Chamomile, German, 69–71
Cinnamon and Cassia,
75–76
Clove, 77
Echinacea, 90–92
Feverfew, 102–4
Ginger, 110–12
Kava-kava, 135–36
Marshmallow, 146–47
Meadowsweet, 148–49
Peppermint, 168–70
Periwinkle, 170–71
Prickly ash, 177–78
Rhubarb, 185–86
Rue, 189
Skunk cabbage, 202–3
Tea tree, 212–13
White willow, 221–22
TRICHOMONIASIS
Goldenseal, 117–18
TRIGLYCERIDES, HIGH
Artichoke, 30–31
Cayenne, 66–68
Fenugreek, 101–2
Garlic, 106–9
Gugul, 122–123
Gymnema, 123–24
Malabar tamarind, 145–46
Oats, 159–60
Onion, 161
Plantain, 175–76
Psyllium, 196–97
Rhubarb, 185–86
Tea, 210–11
Turmeric, 215–16
Wild yam, 223–24
Yucca, 233
TUBERCULOSIS
Aloes, 29
Ashwaganda, 31–32
Chaparral, 71
Chickweed, 73
Echinacea, 90–92
Elecampane, 93–94
Fenugreek, 101–2
Fo-ti, 105

Garlic, 106–9
Ginkgo, 112–14
Ginseng, Oriental, 115–16
Goldenrod, 116–17
Goldenseal, 117–18
Gotu kola, 119–20
Hops, 126–27
Horsetail, 130
Licorice, 140–43
Mullein, 153–54
Red clover, 182–84
Sage, 190–91
Yellow dock, 228–29
Yerba santa, 230–31
TUMOR GROWTH
Aloes, 29
Artichoke, 30–31
Ashwaganda, 31–32
Boneset, 49
Broom, 52–53
Burdock, 56
Calendula, 58–59
Fo-ti, 105
Hydrangea, 131
Lemon balm, 139–40
Mistletoe, 151–52
Mullein, 153–54
Papaya, 163–64
Parsley, 164–65
Shepherd's purse, 200–1
TYPHOID
Boldo, 48
TYPHUS
Garlic, 106–9

U

ULCERS (*SEE ALSO* **MOUTH**
ULCERS)
Alfalfa, 27–28
Aloe, 28
Aloes, 29
Ashwaganda, 31–32
Astragalus, 32–33
Bayberry, 34
Bilberry, 37
Burdock, 56
Cat's claw, 65–66
Chamomile, German, 69–71
Chickweed, 73
Cinnamon and Cassia,
75–76

INDEX

Underscored page references indicate boxed text.

A

A-bisabolol, 70
Absinthin, 227
ACE, 125
Acesulfane-K, 206
Acetaminophen, 74
Acetylcholine, 86, 190
Acetylsalicylic acid, 221
Achillea millefolium (yarrow),
      227–28
Acyclovir, 67, 139
Adaptogen, 115–16, 198
Adenosine 3´,5´-
      monophosphate
      (AMP), 80
Adrenal hormones, 142
Adrenaline, 30
Aescin, 128
Aesculetin, 43
Aesculin, 128
Aesculus hippocastanum (horse
      chestnut), 127–28, 188,
      189
African cherry, 180–81
Agathosma betulina (buchu),
      53–54
Agroforestry Center, 181
ALA, 104
Alanine, 180
Alantolactone, 93
Alder buckthorn (*Frangula
      alnus*), 63

Aldose reductase inhibitors,
      65
Alfalfa (*Medicago sativa*),
      27–28
Allantoin, 82, 176
Allicin, 107
Allium cepa (onion), 161
Allium sativum (garlic),
      106–9, 161
Allopurinol, 69
Aloe (*Aloe vera*), 28–29
Aloes, 29, 199
Aloe vera (aloe), 28–29
Alpha-hydroxy acid,
      173–74
Alpha-linolenic acid (ALA),
      104
Alpha-pinene, 30
Alprazolam, 109
Althaea officinalis
      (marshmallow), 146–47
Amanita phalloides (death cap
      mushroom), 150
Amaranth, 208
American angelica (*Angelica
      atropurpurea*), 88
American Botanical Council,
      4
American ginseng (*Panax
      quinquefolius*), 115
American Herbal Products
      Association, 81–82
Amitriptyline, 109

AMP, 80
Anabsinthin, 227
Ananas comosus (pineapple),
      111, 173–75
Anaphylactic reaction, 54
Anemopsis californica (yerba
      mansa), 229–30
Anethole, 30
Angelica acutiloba (Japanese
      angelica), 88
Angelica archangelica
      (European angelica), 88
Angelica atropurpurea
      (American angelica), 88
Angelica sinensis (dong quai),
      88–89
Angiogenesis, 204
Angiotensin converting
      enzyme (ACE), 125
Anise (*Pimpinella anisum*),
      29–30
Annual wormwood, 209–10
Antabuse, 137
Antacids, 142
Anthemis nobilis (Roman
      chamomile), 69
Anthocyanosides, 37, 46
Anthraquinones, 29, 63, 186,
      199, 229
Antibacterial compounds, 34
Antibiotics, 82, 84, 175
Anticholinergic compounds,
      36

U

Ulmus rubra (slippery elm),
203–4
Uncaria tomentosa (cat's claw),
65–66
Ursolic acid, 132
Urtica dioica (nettle), 7, 126,
157–58
U.S. Department of
Agriculture (USDA),
3–4, 6, 191
U.S. Pharmacopeia, 35, 100,
193, 220
Uva ursi (Arctostaphylos
uva-ursi), 35, 46

V

Vaccinium angusti; V. folia; V.
corymbosum (blueberry),
46, 54
Vaccinium macrocarpum
(cranberry), 46, 84
Vaccinium myrtillus (bilberry),
37, 46
Valepotriates, 218
Valeranone, 215
Valerian (Valeriana officinalis),
217–18
Valium, 11, 109, 135, 167, 218
Venus's-flytrap (Dionaea
muscipula), 7, 208
Verapamil, 103
Verbascum, various species
(mullein), 153–54
Vervain (Verbena officinalis),
219
Viadent, 45
Viagra, 114, 153, 231
Viburnum prunifolium (black
haw), 42–43
Vicks cough drops, 223
Vicks VapoRub, 96
Vincamine, 171
Vinca minor (periwinkle),
170–71

Violets, 189
Violet willow (Salix
daphnoides), 221
Viscum album (mistletoe),
151–52
Vitamin A, 86
Vitamin C, 65, 86, 121,
186–87, 211, 214
Vitamin E, 65, 121, 211
Vitex agnus-castus
(chasteberry),
72–73
Vitexin, 125
Vitexin-rhamnoside,
125
Vitis vinefera (Grape or grape
seed), 120–21
Vomitwort, 144

W

Warfarin, 164
Watermint, 169
Wax myrtle, 34
White horehound (Marrubium
vulgare), 220
White willow (Salix alba), 148,
221–22
Wild chamomile, 69–71
Wild cherry (Prunus serotina),
222–23
Wild yam (Dioscorea villosa),
223–24
Willow. See White willow
(Salix alba)
Witch hazel (Hamamelis
virginiana), 224–25
Withania somniferum
(ashwaganda), 31–32
Withanolides, 31
Wood betony (Stachys
officinalis), 225–26
Wormseed, 48
Wormweed, 209–10
Wormwood (Artemisia
absinthium), 226–27. See
also Annual wormwood

X

Xanax, 109

Y

Yarrow (Achillea millefolium),
227–28
Yellow dock (Rumex crispus),
228–29
Yerba mansa (Anemopsis
californica), 229–30
Yerba santa (Eriodictyon
californicum), 230–31
Yew, 6
Yocon, 232
Yohimbe (Pausinystalia
johimbe), 231–32
Yohimbine, 231–32
Yohimbine hydrochloride, 232
Yohimex, 232
Yucca (Yucca, various species),
233

Z

Zanamivir, 92
Zantac, 142
Zanthoxylum, various species
(prickly ash), 177–78,
183
Zanthoxylum americanum
(northern prickly ash),
177
Zanthoxylum clava-herculis
(southern prickly ash),
177
Zea mays (corn silk), 83
Zedoary (Curcuma zedoaria),
215, 234–35
Zingibain, 111, 174
Zingiber officinale (ginger),
110–12, 174, 215
Zocor, 108
Zoloft, 192
Zostrix, 67
Zovirax, 67, 139